MILLENNIAL #EATS

MILLENNIAL #EATS

THE GENERATION REDEFINING
THE FOOD INDUSTRY

SOPHIE BENSON

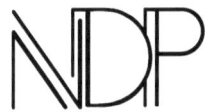

NEW DEGREE PRESS

MILLENNIAL #EATS

The Generation Redefining the Food Industry

ISBN   978-1-64137-086-8   *Paperback*

         978-1-64137-087-5   *Ebook*

I'd like to dedicate this book to all of my fellow food loving, recipe testing, farmer's market frequenting, restaurant trolling Millennials. If there's one I've learned from writing this book, it's that there is a reason we can't seem to stop talking, writing, and reading about food. As the newest wave of consumers, entrepreneurs, marketers, and restaurant managers, we have the power to fundamentally change our country's food culture for the better. The first step is to own our passion for food. I hope that this book inspires your inner foodie and encourages you to never stop fighting for real food.

CONTENTS

INTRODUCTION 11

PART I

MILLENNIALS: WHO WE ARE AND WHY WE CARE
ABOUT FOOD 29

HOW WE GOT HERE: A HISTORY OF THE AMERICAN DIET 43

THE CURRENT STATE OF THE FOOD INDUSTRY AND
HOW MILLENNIALS ARE BEGINNING TO CHANGE IT 55

PART II

THE INTERSECTION OF FOOD AND TECHNOLOGY 67

SOCIAL MEDIA: A POWERFUL VOICE 79

OUR FOOD GURUS: THE PEOPLE WE LISTEN TO,
KNOW, AND TRUST 91

THE INSPIRATION: ENTREPRENEURS IN FOOD 103

PART III

FADS VERSUS TRENDS 121

NOOTROPICS 133

LIQUID NUTRITION 153

KITCHEN STAPLES 167

PARTING WORDS 187

ACKNOWLEDGEMENTS 191

WORKS CITED 193

FEATURED FOODIES 203

"Se nourrir est un besoin. Savoir manger est un art."

"Finding sustenance is a basic need.
Knowing how to eat well is an art."

—FRANÇOIS RABELAIS

INTRODUCTION

———

"Millionaire to millennials: Stop buying avocado toast if you want to buy a home," tweeted *Time* magazine in the spring of May 2017.

According to Australian millionaire Tim Gurner, millennials are facing severe financial problems because of their excessive spending on trendy foods. "When I was trying to buy my first home, I wasn't buying smashed avocado for $19 and four coffees at $4 each," he scoffed in an interview with *60 Minutes*.

Ouch. Whereas I usually tend to brush off the seemingly endless criticism that millennials face nowadays, this comment crept under my skin. I felt personally afflicted by his statement, but not because of the generational criticism. As someone who regularly gets lumped into the millennial generation herself,

I am used to the media roasting us for our self-indulgent, spoiled, entitled nature, and I tend to deflect those criticisms, choosing to believe they don't necessarily apply to me. I did take offense, however, to his condemnation of our spending on food because I knew in that case, I was no exception.

My obsession with and resulting expenditure on food has become a family joke. Every time I come home from college, my first stop is to the grocery store, where I head straight for the organic aisle and proceed to buy all of the nut butters, avocados, bananas, chia seeds, and kale that I can't fathom how my family lives without.

"Holy smokes, Sophie!" I remember my mom saying with disbelief, her mouth agape as she held up the receipt from one of my grocery store trips. She had sent me to pick up a few ingredients for the night's dinner.

"I had to stock up on the essentials!" was all I could muster, shrugging my shoulders and pushing up my eyebrows sheepishly. It was a lame excuse, and I knew it.

My mom was stunned by my purchases of $13 peanut butter and $8 granola, and she had a right to be. The money I am willing to spend on food shocks even me. Why would a college student who lacks any significant source of income spend so excessively on groceries? But the thing was, I knew I wasn't the only one. If *I* was obsessed with food, then so were my friends, and I wanted to figure out why.

As dubious as she once was, my mom has come to accept and even participate in my passion with healthy food and rising trends. For my past two birthdays, she has given me a NutriBullet blender and a Cuisinart food blender. My dad treated me to a ceramic dripper for making pour-over coffee and an individual grinder so that I can freshly grind my coffee beans every morning. I recently purchased myself a tin of stoneground Japanese matcha powder. And what did I put on my Christmas list this year? A gift card to a fresh-pressed juice company.

I'll be the first to admit it: I sound completely food-crazy. Somehow, I had transformed from a high school athlete who lived off of Skippy peanut butter-banana sandwiches to someone who enthusiastically followed the latest food trends, ingredients, and brand names on social media and the Internet. I had grown up on fluffernutters and sugary cereals like any other American kid, yet now, here I am, fastidiously reading nutrition labels, buying organic fruits and vegetables, eating sunflower butter, and roasting veggies in my spare time so that I have healthy meals prepped for the week. When did I start to care so much about what I ate and the food I bought? Why were my friends and I so dedicated to trying the newest, hippest restaurants, going to farmers' markets, and testing recipes? In answering these questions about myself, I made some important discoveries about my whole generation and what its relationship to food says about our future.

Though they may have begun among us millennials, these food trends are spreading across age groups. In his article on millennials leading shifts in the food scene, Brian Boyle explains, "There is certainly enough evidence out there to credit the inertia behind these changes in behavior to the younger generations, and their powerful preferences are permeating through to older generations." Over the past few years, I have introduced my mom to green smoothies, Justin's chocolate peanut butter cups, and almond butter. I've gotten my dad hooked on chia seeds (he claims they are going to make him the next Superman). And my two younger sisters? They now drag my parents straight to the organic aisle of the grocery store.

As much as I'd like to take all the credit for introducing my family to new products, encouraging them to read their food labels more closely, and enlightening them about what they are putting into their bodies, it's clear these food trends are widespread and growing rapidly. I wanted to understand why. Why does my entire generation seem to have become obsessed with food? What instigated this dominance of food in our personal and social lives? Why am I suddenly chatting with my closest friends about what they made for dinner last night, or what they thought of the food at Rose's Luxury (a DC restaurant that typically involves waiting in line for at least a few hours to get a table), or what recipes they want to try this week? And why our generation? Although millennials' new ideas about food are beginning to diffuse into other age groups, our fascination with food clearly isn't evenly distributed across generations.

My seventy-two-year-old grandfather, who remains content with his diet of white bread, fried eggs, sausage, and little to nothing of anything green, is the perfect example of that. "When some people start messing with basic foods . . . quinoa, kale, this and that, it does nothing but ruin food," he told me, as we mulled over the latest food trends at his kitchen table in Vermont. According to him, millennials make the mistake of trying to make food too fancy, whereas his generation just likes to take basic food and make it really good (or so he claims). Funnily enough, his doctor teases him for having a "seventies diet," and the foods he likes to claim as "basic" contain far more preservatives, additives, and sodium than what I try to consume on a regular basis.

Similarly, my dad has always loved and continues to love good food, but he remains uninterested by the newfangled fads and trends that are constantly popping up in the market. Whenever I'm around, he will mispronounce "kombucha" on purpose, crack jokes about my "superfood" chia pudding, or tease me about my love of the organic natural foods section of Stop & Shop.

So what was it about millennials and Generation Yers that caused us to be so preoccupied with all of the newest food trends? I was tired of millennials getting such a bad rap. I wanted to understand why our attitudes toward food seemed to attract so much criticism. But more than that, I wanted to be able to explain and defend my generation's decisions. I wanted to show my dad that these food trends are important and be able to tell him why.

To start, I had to try and understand his perspective. No one denies the major shifts that millennials are causing in the food industry, but like my dad, not everyone believes they are good. Chefs like Anthony Bourdain criticize groups of young foodies who hover over their plates to take photos of their food for Instagram. Restaurant managers worry that the increase in food delivery and food on-the-go is diminishing hospitality and the restaurant experience. Millennials have been accused of increasing food waste because they will purchase food to post it on social media, but never actually eat it.

Certain psychologists and nutritionists worry that the increased adherence to diets like veganism, locavorism, paleo, and gluten-free represents new forms of disordered eating.[1] And baby boomers criticize millennials' absurd spending on food, given that the Boomers restricted themselves to eating out only a few times a month. "It belies reality," millennial food consultant Eve Turow Paul writes in her book, *A Taste of Generation Yum.* "A generation who graduated or is soon to graduate into a landscape of unemployment and low wages eats out at expensive restaurants more than our Baby Boomer or Gen X counterparts, and purchases organic apples and artisanal bread with money that could have gone to laundry." I had to wonder, is our obsession with food unhealthy, or could there be a highly rational justification behind the relationship between millennials and their food?

Ironically, Tim Gurner pointed me toward my answer. In the same interview where he criticized millennials for spending too much money on avocado toast, he actually made an important point, just not in the way he intended. "We're at a point now where the expectations of younger people are very, very high," Gurner stated, attempting to demonstrate the unwarranted sense of entitlement that seems to permeate

---

1   Diet definitions

Veganism: the practice of refraining from consuming animal products, such as meat, eggs, dairy-products and other meat-derived substances.

Locavorism: A movement of people who make a conscious effort to eat food that is grown relatively close to the place of sale and preparation.

The Paleo diet: A diet based on the types of foods eaten by early humans, primarily consisting of meat, fish, vegetables, fruit, and excluding dairy or grain products.

Gluten-free diet: A diet that strictly excludes gluten, a mixture of proteins found in wheat and related grains, including barley, rye, and oat.

the millennial generation. But while the high expectations of millennials may be misguided in the housing, travel, or job markets, they are not only long overdue but also absolutely necessary in the food industry, given its high level of corruption.

What Gurner, Gen Xers, and Baby Boomers may view as irresponsible spending on a food fad or as a superficial, image-based obsession with food is, in reality, symptomatic of deeper convictions among millennials who are finally noticing the rampant corruption of the food system. Rather than accepting it or playing into the hands of food giants and marketing gurus, they are demanding change.

Why are millennials eating so much avocado toast? Because they have realized avocadoes are an accessible, versatile food that is chock-full of nutrients like healthy fats, fiber, potassium, and vitamins. Why are millennials buying more local foods at farm-to-table restaurants and farmers' markets? Because they have realized that the industrialized American food system is corrupt, that giant food companies profit most from the most highly processed foods, and that their local farms can offer fresher, cleaner, more trustworthy products.

These changing attitudes are pushing food giants to purchase smaller, start-up food labels due to the demand from their younger consumers. This is decreasing their monopolistic ability to promote and push only the cheapest, most processed foods and giving more power to small, local businesses and farmers. Furthermore, a new wave of millennials is choosing to give up corporate jobs to go into farming and sustainable agriculture or to start their own food businesses.

Younger consumers are no longer persuaded of health benefits by the labels "lite," "low-fat", or "reduced sugar," so that even the superficiality of the anti-fat, anti-carb weight loss industry is beginning to lose its allure. They're also turning out to be some of the healthiest eaters of any generation, making up 52 percent of organic consumers and eating 52 percent more vegetables than previous generations. They want to know where and whom their food comes from, how it was produced, and what ingredients it contains. Millennials are the most skeptical generation of the food industry, and by combining that skepticism with the market power of consumer demand, they have sparked a food revolution.

In his documentary *In Defense of Food*, Michael Pollan attributes the skewed perceptions of health of the previous generations to nutritionism. "Nutritionism," he says, "is what the food industry uses to show us all the bad things they've taken out and all the good things they've added," which detracts from the true value of food. Food should be understood as a whole entity, not just the sum of its nutrient parts. Pollan says of nutritionism, "It divides the world into good and evil. The blessed are omega 3s, vitamin C, and antioxidants, while the evil is high-fructose corn syrup, saturated fat, and corn syrup."

On the surface, it all sounds true. We're taught to avoid foods with high quantities of high-fructose corn syrup and to eat fatty fish for its omega 3s or to drink a glass of red wine at dinner for its antioxidants. But the problem is, foods can't simply be reduced to their combination of nutrients. The definitions of good and evil around food change all the time. People used to abhor protein because they thought it caused constipation, yet now everyone is working furiously to incorporate protein into their diets. The Kellogg brothers achieved success with their corn flake cereal because they thought carbs were the answer. Now we are taught to reduce our carb intake. The problem with fearing certain foods and adoring others is that marketers can exploit these trends either way.

The food industry's first priority has always been its own bottom line, and to make things worse, giant food processors make the greatest profits from the most highly processed foods. This explains why the Western diet has evolved into meat, white flour, vegetable oils and sugar. "It's cheap, convenient, and processed to taste good," explains Pollan.

One of the biggest events in the history of the American food industry was the construction of the national highway system after World War II. "Once that was built, food processors like Oscar Mayer became really big. And then there was the rise of McDonald's and other hamburger chains along these highways," explains Bruce Kraig, a professor of history at Roosevelt University and president of the Culinary Historians of Chicago.

Newly advertised cans, packages, and pouches became the norm. Canned soup and TV dinners dominated the food market. Previous generations grew up eating meatloaf, potatoes, and macaroni and cheese. The base of their salads was iceberg lettuce. They added salt to already salty food and added sugar to sugary cereals. Their kitchen staples included Hamburger Helper, Spam, and Wonder Bread. This explains why four of the top ten causes of death in the US are chronic diseases linked to diet, such as heart disease, cancer, stroke, and diabetes. It's why the percent of Americans with type 2 diabetes has more than tripled since 2005. It's why over a third of American adults are obese. The transportation system that facilitated the mass distribution of processed foods may have benefited the food industry, but it certainly did not benefit the health of American consumers, small farms, or the environment.

That said, it's no wonder that millennials, who have increased access to technology, to health and nutrition information, and to different foods in general, are beginning to question the food system that has resulted in such high rates of chronic disease linked to diet. Their craving for whole, healthy, unprocessed foods is a reaction against the foods of their parents and grandparents' generation. Similarly, it's no wonder that Baby Boomers and other older generations are defensive of the lifestyles they grew up in and critical of the seemingly unwarranted high expectations of millennials. "The people that own homes today worked very, very hard for it, saved every dollar, did everything they could to get up the property investment ladder," Tim Gurner states, accusing millennials of not understanding the hard work it takes to own property. But his statement begs the question, why shouldn't millennials have it all? Is it really impossible to have both good, clean food and a mortgage, or is that just what the American food industry would like us to believe?

This book deconstructs food fads and trends to reveal their roles in the larger movement that is the millennial approach to food. It reveals why some of the food fads—avocado toast, acai bowls, matcha lattes—that seem to garner the harshest criticism and invite the most mockery actually represent the larger values—buying organic, eating local, looking for functional foods—that are reforming America's food system. A deeper look into some of the most popular food trends over the last few years will provide insight into what consumers are looking for, where the food industry is heading, and what attributes make a food trend stick.

I flesh out the differences between a food trend and a food fad and dive in to some of the movements that are currently taking the food industry by storm, including technology, sustainable agriculture and local-sourcing, the changing relationship between a company and its consumer, and the evolution of our relationship with and perception of our food.

You'll hear the story of kale's rise to fame, of the cofounder of a leading kombucha brand who started brewing the fermented tea as a hair loss product, of how chickpeas achieved market ubiquity, of how one man revolutionized the food scene in Washington, DC, and of several entrepreneurs who ditched finance for the food industry. By the end, you'll have an idea of how millennials and younger consumers are shaping the food industry now as well as how it will continue to evolve in the future.

Be prepared for some commentary from a millennial author herself, replete with personal stories, some blatantly terrible food puns, and my opinions on, well, pretty much everything. Finally, I offer you the Benson Food Longevity Rating scale, or the "BFLR method," a useful tool you can apply in deciding whether to incorporate future food trends into your own diet. I'll help you decide whether you're a fanatic or a skeptic of Bulletproof coffee, whether you should invest in collagen supplements and a matcha whisk, and whether sriracha and kale should become staples in your pantry.

Regardless of your place in the food industry—whether you're the manager of a restaurant who wants to stay up to date on the latest food trends, a marketer who wants to better understand the needs and desires of millennial consumers, or a millennial or Gen Yer yourself, who, like me, was simultaneously baffled and fascinated by the food obsession that seems to have taken over our generation—this book is for you.

Over the past few months, I've read relentlessly about different food trends, food fads, new diets, new technologies in food, up-and-coming companies. I've spoken with marketers of consumer packaged goods, food entrepreneurs, food trend researchers, and foodie Instagram influencers. You will hear from Eve Turow Paul, a self-proclaimed millennial food consultant, a woman who has made a career out of studying the relationship between Millennials and food. Mike Kostyo, Publications Manager at Datassential, one of the largest food market research companies in the US, will explain how food trends are born and how they are sustained. He will shed light on the various definitions of "healthy" that have evolved over the course of different generations.

You will gain an understanding of the Instagram strategies behind some of the most famous food-based influencers, as well as the stories behind their greatest successes and biggest failures. Dave Stever, the charismatic employee who worked his way from tour guide at the Ben & Jerry's factory to Chief

Marketing Officer of the company, will describe what creates a successful connection between a company and its customers. Brett Schulman, the CEO of Cava restaurants, offers his perspective on how technology is changing the food industry. And Cullen Gilchrist, the cofounder of Union Kitchen, DC's first food incubator gives his advice to budding food entrepreneurs. All of this will be presented through the lens of a self-proclaimed, food-loving millennial.

I had initially started out blindly, wanting nothing more than simply to understand why millennials and members of Gen Y had become so fixated on food, how we got here, and where we are going. I wasn't sure if I would come out another pessimistic critic of my own generation or a champion of the millennial food movement. But the more people I spoke to, the more inspired I became by young entrepreneurs in food. The more research I did, the more strongly I felt that our reaction against so much of the traditionally processed foods that the commercial food industry bombards us with is completely justified. Don't get me wrong, I remain a skeptic of many fads that have recently been hyped up—gluten-free diets, Bulletproof coffee, and health food bloggers to name a few. But all in all, I believe our generation is moving the food industry in the right direction—toward food that is humanely produced and beneficial to both our bodies and our environment. I believe that millennials are the twenty-first century revolutionaries of the food industry.

I understand why Tim Gurner targeted millennials for their consumption of avocado toast. On the surface, the zeal with which we seem to throw ourselves into new food trends can appear bizarre, careless, or overly indulgent. But the Australian millionaire along with all the other millennial critics, failed to step back and ask, why avocado toast? From a millennial's perspective, it's an accessible, affordable, versatile, DIY meal that checks multiple nutritional boxes. Our decision to spend money on high-quality, clean, whole foods like avocado on whole-wheat bread is a means of taking back control of our health, our lives, and of the food industry itself. So the next time my dad purposely mispronounces kombucha, pokes fun at my latest food combination, or teases me about my stereotypically millennial order at a restaurant, I think I'll just ask him if he would like a side of avocado toast to go with his attitude.

PART I

THE FUTURE OF FOOD

CHAPTER 1

MILLENNIALS: WHO WE ARE AND WHY WE CARE ABOUT FOOD

———

Eve Turow Paul, the self-professed sole millennial food consultant to date, and therefore an expert on the subject, titled her book *A Taste of Generation Yum*. When I asked her about the term's origin, her response was adamant: "There should be a name for it," she answered simply. "Over 50 percent of the millennial population, and over 50 percent of Generation Z consider themselves to be foodies. Generation Yum is that cohort of foodies, and when you break it down, that's over a quarter of the population of the *world*."

She coined the term Generation Yum to represent that entire

population of food-obsessed young people. These people are the ones I want to explore and understand, the people this book is about. In order to explain the rising frequency and variety of food trends occurring within my generation, I needed to first understand our relationship with food and determine where our passion for food originated.

Sitting in my cubicle at work these days, I listen to fellow colleagues describe what they have brought for lunch that day, what new restaurant their significant other is taking them to this weekend, or what new food combination they have recently tried. I even heard a young woman at the desk over ask around for new nut substitute recommendations. "I'm just getting *so* sick of almonds," she lamented to her fellow food-fanatic colleagues.

I participate in food dialogue as much as the rest of my generation, but I couldn't seem to let go of this nagging feeling that the dominance of food in our daily lives and our obsession with food in day-to-day conversation had to be unhealthy to a certain extent. While sometimes I find myself seriously craving one particular food item or meal, more recently, I have found myself experiencing a kind of apathy toward food.

It's almost as if the constant bombardment of new foods and recipes within the media, on social media apps, and among the people I am surrounded by has overwhelmed me. I have so many options available to me that no particular one stands out. I've lost my ability to listen to what my body is craving. And I'm not the only one; the young people of Generation Yum no longer rely on our bodies to tell us what we need or are craving because the image culture surrounding food has exploded, leaving us with an absurd surplus of options. Instagram influencers tell us which new crazy food fad we should try, lifestyle bloggers and nutritionists post the healthy recipes we should be eating, and our newspapers send us recipes of the day. I no longer cook based on what I am craving, but on the new ingredient or recipe I want to try.

My conversation with Christopher Myers, a man who has spent the last forty years in the restaurant industry, heightened my skepticism of my generation's enthusiasm for food in another way. "People want to eat healthier . . . or at least they think they do," he told me. As someone who co-owns seven Flour Bakeries in Boston with his wife, Joanne Chang, Christopher sees that despite the new emphasis on healthy foods, people continue to indulge their sweet tooths. He noted that Flour's vegan and gluten-free baked goods, even though they taste every bit as delicious and interesting as the full-sugar pastries, make up the rock bottom of their sales. "There's just not as big a market for it, or if there is, they're not coming to Flour for that."

As I mused over his anecdote, I couldn't help but wonder if

this massive trend toward healthier food could be a sham. The challenge our society is currently facing, or the "cross-hairs" as Christopher called it, is that people want to eat food that's really flavorful but that's also really good for you. Mike Kostyo, Publications Manager at the food market research firm, Datassential, had some research to back him up.

Datassential had conducted a survey in which they asked each participant what they had eaten over the past twenty-four hours. People cited extremely high percentages of vegetables and fresh produce and low percentages of things like snacks and potato chips in their responses. But when Datassential conducted another study requiring participants to keep diaries of what they actually ate, the results were the exact opposite. "Both of those data points are helpful and interesting," Mike says. "People have aspirational ideas of what they're eating that don't match what they're actually eating."

One of his jobs at Datassential is to help consumers find foods that are good for them, but still retain the satisfying qualities of, say, a crunchy potato chip or a gooey homemade cookie. I wondered whether the trends among young foodies toward healthier foods were resolute and sustainable or just another "fad" effort to eat healthy that rarely amounts to real change. The evolution of food throughout previous generations has left the relationship between millennials and our food nothing less than complicated.

Now, more than ever before, food is a symbol of social status. "Sometimes certain foods achieve a status beyond what their physical nutritional attributes are, and they become symbols," explains David Sax, author of *The Tastemakers: Why We're Crazy for Cupcakes but Fed Up with Fondue*. "Something edible transforms into something cultural." Numerous psychologists and experts in the food industry discuss the newfound use of food as social signaling. Certain foods now represent aspects of class, identity, and politics. Posting food on social media is a method of signaling both privilege and access to various resources such as time, money, knowledge of where to go, and the ability to find unique, trendy food items.

"Food is not just what you're eating. Today, food is a branding statement. People are not eating stunt foods for themselves; they're eating them as an act of branding or performance," Eve states. These people use images to signal a wide variety of things: to show off a new recipe, to receive feedback, to prove that they are environmentally conscious, that they are foodies, that they are healthy, or that they are in-the-know about the food scene. No one is buying the decadent cookie-candy ice cream sundaes with caramel drizzle on top because they think it's going to make them feel good; they are using them to enhance their personal brand. Similarly, no one posts the leftovers they found in the back of their fridge or the bowl of instant ramen noodles they ate while cramming for a midterm, because social media has allowed us to post only the carefully curated, elaborate, photogenic foods that we have either purchased or made at home. Food has become an accessory of our identities because we can now carefully craft the presentation of certain ingredients or dishes to create a very specific image of ourselves. It's no wonder then that these images have created ridiculously high standards of how, where, and what we eat.

"My top learning is that millennials still lead the pack as the most anxious, most stressed out, and loneliest generation," Eve told me over the phone. Social media has become such an integral part of the daily lives of millennials, and so Facebook, Instagram, and Twitter are influencing food and hunger cues more than our bodies. Various forms of disordered eating have appeared and expanded within the millennial generation.

Orthorexia, a fear of food, is one that has gained ground over the past few years, as more and more people choose to partic-ipate in non-medically recommended elimination diets like Whole30, the Paleo diet, and veganism. The term "elimination diet" on its own is a vague concept. Medically, it is used to describe the process of eliminating foods from one's diet in hopes of ascertaining the root causes of digestive problems or discomfort. It typically only requires the temporary elimi-nation foods and allows patients to slowly reintroduce foods back into their diets. However, when used in the context of self-selected diets, it can also represent unhealthy attitudes or decisions regarding food.

"Anything that promotes an emphasis on what something looks like rather than how it makes you feel is probably going to be detrimental to body image and take away from eating mindfully," Dr. Sarah Bellovin Goldman, a psychologist at Georgetown University, explained, referencing strict elimination diets in particular. "Any time you are creating a diet or a particular set of foods you're supposed to eat, you're not listening to your body." This phenomenon occurs among people who choose to follow a form of elimination diet, like carb-free, gluten-free, sugar-free, etc., not for medical reasons, but out of personal preference and often the desire to lose weight.

While the diets aren't necessarily forms of disordered eating in themselves, they have the potential to be harmful because of the psychological implications surrounding eating and because they are often examples of people restricting their diets in a certain way to assert control over something in their lives. Sarah suggests that any rules surrounding food have the potential to be harmful. As someone who works with clients who often have histories of eating disorders, she finds that on the surface, her clients may appear to have solid reasoning behind the pursuit of an elimination diet, but on a deeper level, the diets are often eating disorders masquerading themselves in a new form. One could argue that restricting yourself from any food is contradictory to the idea of listening to your body. She encourages her clients to think of the slogan, "rules break, guidelines bend." Often rules are too rigid, whereas guidelines can still fit into the idea of moderation and intuitive eating.

Rules also tend to intensify the perceptions of good and bad we attach to our own diets. The added pressure stemming from food accounts on social media—both those who post only the healthiest meals and those who post the most indulgent—creates further confusion and stress in our lives about what we should be eating. Sarah explained that there has been a historical "all or nothing and feast or famine" relationship with food in Western culture, adding that we tend to attach morality to our diets as well.

We all bear witness to it in our own lives. People are constantly saying things like, "I was good today. I ate so much salad!" or, "I was so bad today." According to Sarah, the language of good and bad that we use around food can be harmful because it makes it harder for people to find a healthy balance in the middle. The majority of the clients she has helped have never even thought about maintaining their weight because they are so focused on changing it. The perception of certain foods as bad or good that is created by both the traditional media channels and the various forms of social media negatively impacts our ability to listen to our internal hunger cues. We focus on what we think we should be eating rather than what our body is actual craving.

In Eve Turow Paul's analysis of new food trends, such as the shift toward locally sourced products and healthier whole foods, and the explosion of diets like veganism, Whole30, and Paleo, she discovered an underlying reason for the spike in adherence to these diets—a desire for control within Generation Yum, or all the young foodies who make up the millennial and Gen Y generations. "Eaters are exerting control over what they eat in very particular ways, and it's a socially acceptable, if not celebrated, practice," she writes.

Eve spoke with Mark Bittman, the iconic American food journalist and author, about the exponential growth of interest in food as a way of counteracting our corrupt food system. Mark acknowledged our generation's frustration with fake, processed foods and the lack of clarity surrounding the origin and production methods behind the foods we put into our bodies. He offered trends like veganism as methods of coping, by "simplifying and regulating your own eating." While Eve agreed that the recent increase in food trends such as gluten-free, vegan, paleo, flexitarianism, and locavorism stems from our mistrust in the food system, she believes a need for control—direct control over what we put into our bodies—is the deeper cause underlying it all.

I pondered Eve's theory as I read Roxane Gay's newest book,

Hunger, which, ironically, details in large part a woman's unhealthy relationship with food. Roxane, who often struggles to grocery shop or cook because she is picky, constantly busy, and always trying to lose weight, admitted that even she found some degree of comfort in cooking. "There is, I must admit, something very satisfying about making things from scratch, to know every dish in a meal was made by your own hands," she writes. Furthermore, as someone who is not a particularly comfortable or experienced chef, she requires clear instructions and guidance from the recipes she uses. She's not the only one.

Although I long to become so adept in the kitchen that I can just throw ingredients together to create a tasty meal or to have made a recipe so many times that I can recreate it from memory, I am a far cry from that level of skill or expertise. There is something satisfying in knowing that as long as you follow the recipe relatively closely, you should end up with something tasty. There's a comfort in the fact that people have used this recipe and crafted this meal with success before you.

So when I read Roxane's words, "What has fascinated me about cooking is how it's actually a really good endeavor for a control freak," I simply had to laugh and agree with her. Perhaps, because there is so little else we seem to be able to control in our lives—the information that companies like Google and Facebook are allowed to amass about us, the ever-increasing presence of technology in our lives, what schools we get into, or even who our president is—perhaps, we are looking to exert what little control we can over the food that we create and put into our bodies.

On the one hand, it sounds perfectly rational. If we can't trust the food system, we must create our own food system by choosing only to intake very specific and restricted foods. On the other hand, it sounds like borderline disordered eating, and I began to wonder if that was what had made me feel so uneasy about my generation's food fanaticism in the first place.

The newest celebrity converts to veganism, including Mark Bittman and Bill Clinton, both highlighted the weight loss they had experienced once they shifted their diets. Gluten-free diets, in their most original form, closely resemble low-carb diets because gluten is predominantly found in things like bread and pasta. Give up carbs like that and you are sure to experience weight loss, at least initially.

What makes these diets any different than following a Weight Watchers program, drinking SlimFast, eating Lean Cuisine, or doing a juice cleanse? Regardless of their methods, all of the above involve restricting your diet in some way and denying your body of certain types of food. We may tout these new trends as environmentally friendly, as a rebuttal of processed foods, or as supportive of local businesses, but what if, at their core, they are all various forms of disordered eating? What if they are just all ways for us to extend some semblance of control over our lives?

Yes, when taken to an extreme, any of these diets can result in adverse health effects. But the thing is, the recent surge in popularity of vegan and Paleo and Whole30 diets is just one facet of the millennial movement toward healthier food. I believe in returning to the consumption of whole foods and eliminating the processed ones. I believe in the local food movement because it offers us cleaner, simpler foods from people we can trust. I'm even a believer in experimenting with new diets and new fads that might pop up. But I am also a huge believer in moderation.

As a generation that is being bombarded, frequently and intensely, with new technologies, new foods, and new companies, it is always in our best interest to be skeptical and to ensure that our obsession with food only goes so far. "You have to look harder to find information that's accurate," warns Carol Day, a certified nutritionist at Georgetown University. "You have to know basic things about how food is produced, and how it's developed by companies to light up pleasure centers in your brain for sugar, salt, and fat. If you don't know that we're living in a capitalist country that manufactures food for profit, not well-being, you're already on the wrong path," she explains. According to her, there's no inherent risk in adhering to veganism, so long as you find out all you can about being vegan and the safety of the food supply.

As for me, I say, "Let them eat vegan!" Whereas elimination diets like veganism and paleo are embraced by the most forward-thinking, risk-taking young foodies and may never expand to the greater US population, the overarching trend toward real, healthy, clean food isn't going anywhere. "Among Gen Z and millennials, people are looking for foods that give them more than calories; they want functional benefits," claims Dave Stever, Chief Marketing Officer at Ben & Jerry's. Millennials are justified in seeking control over their food because for so long American consumers have been victims of the food industry.

While previous generations have succumbed to the wealth and the power of food giants like McDonald's and Coca-Cola, increasing their consumption of highly processed foods with high salt, sugar, and fat content, millennials are refusing to do so. Their craving for whole, unprocessed food that comes from honest companies is a direct backlash against the high degree of corruption and processing that occurs within the food industry. Critics may find food trends like avocado toast and acai bowls easy to mock, but they are missing the point. Those creations are just rungs on the ladder of our progress toward creating food that is both tasty and nutritious. For once, millennials are justified in their idealism. In order to achieve the generation that both provides and consumes sustainable, clean, whole, and delicious food, we have to believe that we can.

CHAPTER 2

HOW WE GOT HERE: A HISTORY OF THE AMERICAN DIET

————

In order to understand the millennial reaction against the unhealthy, highly processed foods that have come to dominate the food market, we have to look at how we got where we are today. Throughout the twentieth century, the food industry evolved a certain way due to a variety of historical events and technological innovations. There is a history of food in the United States that explains why the rates of obesity among white American males have increased from under 5 percent in 1982 to anywhere from 25 to 45 percent today, depending on age. That history explains why higher rates of obesity are linked to industrialized, affluent nations. It explains why the number of heart attacks and cases of diabetes has increased along with the obesity epidemic. It explains why Americans eat highly processed junk foods because even as our knowledge of nutrition has increased, food companies have only gotten better at manipulating that knowledge for their own purposes. They have only gotten better at manipulating government regulations and wielding their wealth and power to increase their own profits.

During the 1930s, when American families were struggling to make ends meet amidst the Great Depression and decreasing their expenditure on food, large food companies wanted to avoid a drop in profits. In 1933, The National Biscuit Company created Ritz crackers and launched the recipe "Mock Apple Pie," which was made almost entirely of Ritz crackers, in order to allow consumers to indulge despite the high apple prices at the time. The same decade witnessed the creation of the epitome of all processed foods—Spam—which had a shelf life of over seven years.

In his article "Dining Through the Decades: 100 Years of American Food," David Leite writes that in 1937, "Hormel pitched in by developing arguably the most indestructible of all comestibles: Spam." Within a matter of years, Spam appeared in the kitchens of almost every American kitchen and became a staple in the diets of the military troops in World War II. "Popular dishes of the period were inexpensive, one-pot meals such as macaroni and cheese, chili, oxtail soup, casseroles, and meat loaf," explains Leite, adding that the only vegetables present in dishes tended to be the cheap ones: carrots, peas, and potatoes. And the people who weren't cooking at home, the urbanites, were living off of cheap street food like hot dogs and hamburgers.

As the thirties became the forties, the food scene didn't have a chance to improve before the arrival of World War II. Families again were forced to ration their food and learn to live off of less. During this decade, the sales of convenience and prepared foods increased. "This is when margarine came in as a replacement for butter," explains Melanie Barnard, a Bon Appétit columnist and author of *Short & Sweet*. But if the thirties and forties were bad, the food scene of the fifties hit rock bottom.

The decade has been called the "nadir of American cuisine." At the heart of that lies the rise of processed foods. During the fifties, the modern-day highway system was created, which allowed for the mass distribution of processed foods. Swanson introduced the ninety-eight-cent TV dinner in 1953, and along with it came canned foods, frozen fish sticks, tuna noodle casserole, and California dip, which was a combination of powder and sour cream.

The American food industry, from the 1930s through the 1950s, relied on consumer demand for pre-packaged, convenient, foods with long shelf lives. The system that evolved during that time period—a modern highway network that facilitated distribution, food companies exploiting consumer desires for their own benefit, and a market that relied heavily on highly processed foods—still exists today.

There lies infinite evidence of the rampant corruption of the food industry, from scandals in the honey business and fraudulent substitutes in the olive oil industry to collusion between major food companies to prohibit healthier food regulations from the government and the convoluted labeling of highly processed items like high-fructose corn syrup. "More of us are wanting to buy the food we know the source of," says Clint Walker, owner of Walker Honey Farm. "The honey industry is perfect for an enlightened food culture." But even honey has been exploited by massive manufacturers that are willing to go to any length to ensure the increase of their profits.

Honey has long been touted as a more natural alternative to white sugar and with the new wave of health-conscious consumers, food manufacturers have been making the switch in products ranging from bread and ham to chips. The honey business is booming because of it. For over a decade, global honey consumption has increased by over $40 million a year, with the United States responsible for half of the world's honey intake.

However, while demand continues to soar, honey production has dropped. Over the past decade, bees have been dying in record numbers. Beekeepers have lost up to 50 percent of their colonies in one year. "The only way to explain that gap," says Norberto Garcia of the International Honey Exporters Association, "is honey adulteration." The culprits are savvy honey producers, particularly the Chinese producers in this case, who cut the pure honey with cheaper substitutes, also known as honey laundering.

Certain syrups and sugars can go undetected by the technology that tests for honey adulteration, such as rice-produced syrups, which the Chinese discovered and proceeded to export to the US at shockingly low prices. This not only put American consumers at risk due to the potential presence of harmful antibiotics, lead, and other various chemicals in Chinese-produced honey, but also suffocated the domestic honey industry.

The surplus of cheap honey on the market pushed American producers out of business, so much so that in 2001, the US government declared that the Chinese were unfairly dumping honey into the US market and imposed heavy, anti-dumping tariffs. But for all the administrative barriers the government may impose, international honey producers continue to find loopholes through ultra-filtration methods that make the honey impossible to trace or by sending it through third countries. Unfortunately, the honey industry is only one of the many food industries riddled with widespread fraud. It happens in the international trade of foods from olive oils and black beans to walnuts and teas.

Peter Laufer, a writer and professor of journalism at the University of Oregon, even became skeptical of the label "organic." He recently noticed two products that he found in his kitchen—some organic black beans from Bolivia and some walnuts supposedly from Kazakhstan. He launched into a full-blown research project to discover where the products came from, but no matter how many people he talked to, he continued to get vague answers. "It seems to me if everything is clean as a whistle, you'd be proud to say where the food came from," he states in the NPR article "Can You Trust That Organic Label On Imported Foods?"

From there, evidence of mislabeling built up to a certain degree. Laufer found that there is an inevitable conflict of interest in the process of organic labeling because the companies that inspect and certify organic farms are paid by those who are being certified. Fortunately, organic labels remain far more trustworthy than other labels like "natural," that have almost no restrictions. Organic farmers do have strict rules to follow and are required to have third-party certifiers inspect their operations. But still, if even the label "organic" begs mistrust, how are we supposed to trust the rest of the food industry?

In a similar vein, the Corn Refiners Association of the US proposed changing the name high-fructose corn syrup to "corn sugar" in 2010. This attempt at renaming was most likely an effort on their behalf to present it as more natural. The problem is that no matter what you label it, high-fructose corn syrup is far from natural. It involves industrial processing that uses a genetically engineered enzyme.

When corn syrup was discovered in the 1960s, it was a golden ticket for the food industry. Corn commodity subsidies made it cheaper than alternative sugars and high-fructose corn syrup has the ability to increase the shelf-life of most foods. In her article for *The Atlantic*, "Don't Sugar-Coat High-Fructose Corn Syrup," Anna Lappé writes, "Relatively cheap, high-fructose corn syrup was a cornerstone of the food industry's super-size-me strategy." So with such a valuable ingredient, it's almost not shocking that the Corn Refiners Association spent between $13 and $20 million on a public relations campaign on the natural goodness of high-fructose corn syrup, particularly targeting mothers. That amount might sound more shocking when you realize that it's nine times what the CDC allocated for its entire five-a-day fruits and vegetables program. What happens when you have a food industry in which the giant food processors hold the wealth and the influence? According to Lappé, "Thanks to these dietary trends and the shift toward a high-fat, high-sugar, highly processed diet, obesity is a national epidemic, and a costly one."

Unfortunately, the corruption of the food industry extends far beyond mislabeling. In some cases, giant food companies manage to squash government regulations before they can even be enacted. In 1977, the US Senate Committee on Nutrition and Human Needs, also known as the McGovern Committee, released a report of dietary goals for the US that included a list of guidelines encouraging lower consumption of animal-based foods and higher consumption of plant-based foods. The guidelines make perfect sense considering that Americans overconsume meat and should, for their health, increase the level of vegetables and whole grains in their diets.

According to Dr. Neal Barnard, the president of the Physicians Committee for Responsible Medicine, "Plant-based diets are the nutritional equivalent of quitting smoking." So, yes, the guidelines almost undoubtedly would have improved the health of American consumers, but because it had the potential to harm the profits of several large food companies, the phrase "decrease meat consumption" was removed entirely from the report due to industry pressure. And it didn't stop there; shortly after the guidelines were released, the entire Senate Nutrition committee was disbanded.

Furthermore, the committee made no mention of scientific research on the health consequences of eating meat, because had it done so, its members would not have been able to justify their removal of the decrease-meat-consumption clause.

Dr. Michael Gregor, a physician and author of *How Not to Die*, found that members of the US Dietary Guidelines advisory committee have financial ties to candy bar companies and organizations such as McDonald's Council on Healthy Lifestyles and Coca-Cola's Beverage Institute for Health and Wellness. These same companies, including Coca-Cola, McDonald's, and even Philip Morris, the cigarette maker, also have ties to the medical world, such as the American Academy of Family Physicians. The extent of the power and influence of these food giants appears endless as they seep into the lives of consumers everywhere from grocery stores to doctors' offices.

In a TED talk at Harvard Law School, Stephan Guyenet explained that the US has seen a radical change from simple, home-cooked food to commercially prepared food over the past two centuries. He identifies some of the major contrasts between the diets of previous generations and American diets today. "In the 1800s," he explains, "most people lived on or near farms, so food was restricted to the seasonal and local crops." But the turn of the nineteenth century brought with it electric refrigerators, the proliferation of grocery stores, the expansion of circulation and storage that allowed for mass food preparation, and the increase in all of these labor-saving technologies.

"You would think people would be cooking more of their own

food," says Guyenet, "but it actually led to the rise of commercially prepared food." He goes on to support his claim with an array of mind-boggling statistics. In 1889, 93 percent of all food spending was on food to be eaten at home. In 2009, food eaten at home only made up 51 percent of total food spending due to a dramatic increase in fast food consumption and eating out. Butter and lard, which were the dominant added fats in the early nineteenth century, were surpassed by the use of margarine, shortening, and oils, which increased total consumption of added fats over the century.

Polyunsaturated fat consumption increased by 300 percent over that time. From 1970 to 2010, the US saw a 20 percent increase in caloric intake, which translates to an increase of roughly 425 calories a day. Technological innovation in glass-blowing made soda cheaper and the invention of vending machines made it more accessible. Cane sugar was replaced by high-fructose corn syrup.

According to Guyenet, "Processed food manufacturers are using extensive engineering of foods to maximize palatability and likelihood of repeat purchase and to minimize production costs." But they're not only engineering food, they're using cultural engineering to drive sales, which manifests itself in the fact that the second most recognizable figure to US children, second only to Santa Claus, is Ronald McDonald. The traditional American diet was simple, minimally refined, and required home preparation. Today, it's hyperpalatable, commercially engineered, high in added sugars, and requires far less effort.

Today, because of the way the American diet has evolved, we face an obesity epidemic in which 40 percent of our country's adults are obese and a whopping 70 percent are either overweight or obese. The top causes of death in our country are linked directly to our diets. So it's no wonder that millennials are fed up with an over-processed, non-nutritious diet and obesity levels that seem be rising with no end in sight. It's no wonder that millennials now base their level of trust in a company on the company's level of transparency across its practices—from business ethics and the impact of food on health and the environment to food safety. Millennials want to see companies include information on product labels, offer engagement opportunities on company websites, and protect any whistleblowers, in order to ensure integrity. It's no wonder that millennials are seeking out local, trustworthy, safe, whole, and healthier foods because they are witnessing the frighteningly harmful results of a lifelong bad diet.

CHAPTER 3

THE CURRENT STATE OF THE FOOD INDUSTRY AND HOW MILLENNIALS ARE BEGINNING TO CHANGE IT

———

"I'd like a large vanilla iced latte with a shot please."

"Our large iced lattes typically come with three shots, so would you like to add one more?" I asked, just to clarify.

The girl looked at me blankly, "Wait, there are espresso shots in that? No one told me that last time."

"So, a latte is made up of espresso shots and milk, and then we add the vanilla flavoring for you," I explained, hoping I had succeeded in masking any sign of irritation or condescension. It was hard for me to understand people who ordered without having a single clue what exactly they were asking for.

Another girl asked me once how many calories were in one of our muffins. "I'm not positive, but I would guess around 400," I told her, having had enough experience with muffins from various coffee shops and with baking in general to give her what I knew was a close estimate. Her jaw dropped, and she immediately chose to buy something else.

As passionate for food as we seem to be, I don't think our generation has quite realized the effort it takes to stay a smart and informed consumer, especially when large food companies now have so much information they can use to manipulate us. Something may read "natural" on the label, but that guarantees approximately nothing. People still assume that yogurt and granola bars are healthier snacks for their kids without realizing that many of those brands load up their products with added sugar. There is no requirement for companies to be able to label their product with the word "natural." And Starbucks may highlight their drinks as low-calorie, but that doesn't mean their skinny vanilla latte is good for you.

"I was at a community farm once, and there was a raised

bed—about 3 feet by 3 feet—that had a sign saying Chipotle on it. I asked what it was for, and the farmers told me Chipotle gets about five tomatoes from us a year. That allows them to put us on our list of where they source their tomatoes," Eve Turow Paul told me. "There is a lot of greenwashing in this industry."[2]

If one thing about the millennial attitude toward food can be justified, it's their distrust of large food corporations and government regulations on food. To name just a few examples, CBS recently came out with a list of "11 Revolting Things Government Lets in Your Food" which included mold and rot, insect eggs and maggots, rodent hair, and animal feces. The FDA allows companies to label their food products with the term "natural" as long as there is nothing artificial or synthetic included in or added to a food—guidelines that simply ignore the food production, processing, or manufacturing methods, such as the use of pesticides, pasteurization, irradiation, and any correlated health effects. They also allow the number of calories to be inaccurate within 20 percent of the product's precise number of calories. So that granola bar that claims it contains 180 calories could contain up to 220. The food industry certainly does not lack ways to fool consumers or get around FDA regulations.

---

2   Greenwashing: Inaccurate information spread by an organization in order to present an environmentally responsible public image.

In many cases, the food industry exploits its knowledge of consumers: our biology, our cost sensitivity, our values, and the media we are constantly exposed to. In his ruthlessly satirical open letter to American consumers, "Dear Consumers, Please Don't Eat Healthfully," Patrick Mustain exposes the questionable ethics of the food industry. He cites the food industry's ability to use its wealth and power to overturn government-mandated standards for advertising foods to children.

In 2009, Congress had commissioned the Interagency Working Group, which included the FTCC, CDC, FDA, and USDA to develop these standards. The guidelines claimed that foods advertised to children must "provide a meaningful contribution to a healthful diet," which meant those items have to contain at least half by weight or more of foods such as fruits, vegetables, whole grains, and lean meat. What was an effort to outline strict guidelines for children's food items—guidelines that would encourage children to eat food that is better for them—was destroyed by the economic power of the food industry. Those guidelines represented a potentially massive drop in their profits as well as a drastic increase in the cost of manufacturing healthier foods, so like clockwork, they used their wealth and influence to force the Working Group to withdraw the guidelines.

Mustain also mentions the biological bias of humans toward salty, sugary, and fatty foods. Because we evolved during a time when food was scarce, our bodies adapted to crave those types of food. While those inborn cravings for sugar, salt, and fat were necessary when famines were common, they have now caused a mismatch between our biology and our environment. Those ingredients light up the same pleasure centers of our brain as cocaine.

The food industry constantly exploits these facts, adding vanilla flavor to baby formula, overloading fruit juices with added sugar, and using corn syrup in unjustifiable quantities in children's snacks. The problem is that government regulations have encouraged the production and use of these ingredients.

The food industry profits the most from its extremely processed foods, opting to grow corn, soybeans, wheat and rice because the government provides subsidies that keep supplies of these crops high and their prices low. "The American farm system has turned into a calorie conveyer belt," says Dr. David Ludwig, the author of *Always Hungry?* This all manifests itself in the fact that the main causes of death in America are chronic diseases related to diet: heart disease, cancer, stroke, and diabetes.

Amid a rather depressing view of the food industry, Michael Pollan implies that we are faced with two choices: "Surrender to the Western diet, junk food, processed food, fast food, and wait for evolution to adapt us to it," which he argues is too expensive, harmful, and unsustainable. Or, "We can take the more practical, more economical, and the more beautiful path, which is simply to change the way we're eating," which Pollan believes is the right way. The thing is, I think millennials are doing that. And they're not just changing the way they're eating; they're changing the way they buy, produce, and manufacture food.

Brett Schulman, CEO of Cava, had a few incredible real-world examples of these changes. One of the most fascinating things Brett mentioned during his interview was that new food and health trends are forcing producers to change because the trends are induced and supported by consumers. He proudly offered three examples of farms that Cava sources from: first, Richardson Farms, which is a third generation kale farm on the East Coast that operates ten months out of the year; second, a shepherd who uses sustainable and ethical practices and who has now taught other co-op farms his practices in order to build a supply chain big enough to support Cava's needs; and third, Dave Oien the CEO and cofounder of Timeless Seeds, who owns an organic lentil farm that practices sustainable agriculture.

The story of Dave Oien is a fascinating one. He grew up in a family of farmers in Conrad, Montana. As he was coming of age, things were just starting to move toward an industrial system, but he was determined not to farm that way, nor was he convinced that it was going to be viable for his family's small, 280-acre farm. After studying both environmental and social change movements throughout college, he returned home and began to experiment with rotational crops. He eventually discovered lentils, which have the capacity to work with bacteria to create their own fertilizer, both for the lentil plant itself and the next crop, so that if you rotate lentils with a grain, the grain yield will be higher the next year as well.

With lentils as the key crop, he developed the company Timeless Seeds in the late eighties with three other local farmers. Today, they rotate up to twenty-one crops and manage to use plants to provide resources for one another that would otherwise require chemicals. It's a million-dollar business that sells to natural food stores all over the country and relies on twenty to thirty growers each year.

Timeless Seeds managed to invent an entirely new farming system and create its own market by connecting to eaters rather than large corporations who control the food chain from beginning to end. Their success is driven by the successful combination of their mission to create more opportunities in sustainable farming, to develop and sell unique, nutritious food products, and to be a socially and environmentally responsible company.

Dave is just one example of the movement toward more

sustainable farming methods. The incredible thing is that millennials are becoming active participants in agriculture. According to the US Department of Agriculture, the number of farmers under thirty-five years old is increasing for only the second time in the last century. And in the same census, it was reported that the number of farmers from ages twenty-five to thirty-four grew 2.2 percent, while other groups of farmers decreased by more than 10 percent.

These young farmers are more likely to grow organically, limit pesticide use, diversify their crops, and involve themselves in their local food systems. In an article on the return of young people to farms, Eve Turow Paul told *The Washington Post*, "I get calls all the time from farmers—some of the largest farmers in the country—asking me when the local and organic fads will be over. It's my pleasure to tell them 'Look at this generation. Get on board or go out of business.'" Our generation isn't only revolutionizing farming methods, but other firms with social missions are turning toward production methods that might appear backward to the traditional businessman.

Ben & Jerry's is another great example. Dave Stever, the company's Chief Marketing Officer, told me that he had learned one of his greatest anti-business lessons from Jerry. Dave was working on testing a new flavor and explained, "As a business you tend to get caught up on the numbers. What's the gross margin? What's the target volume? What's the price point?"

Well, as they were tasting in the lab one day, Jerry happened to walk by and Dave waved him in. As Jerry tasted the new flavor, Dave explained that they were struggling to figure out how to price this flavor correctly so that they could meet their profit margin. Jerry started laughing at him: "Ben and I never worried about this stuff. We didn't worry about what we were going to price things at or what the margin was. We just tried to make the best product we could and then we figured out the rest of the stuff along the way."

Dave took that same product line and decided to make it the best they possibly could before they priced it, working backward in a way from a business standpoint. "It was a good reminder of why you do this stuff," Dave said. "You do it for the love of ice cream. You don't do it to hit a margin or a price point. You're trying to make the best thing you can, so your fans get it and love it."

Jerry's lesson seems to be trickling down throughout food companies that are aiming to please millennials, who expect not only high-quality products but companies that uphold commitments to corporate social responsibility, safe production methods, and fresh, clean ingredients.

PART II

THE PEOPLE BEHIND THE TRENDS

CHAPTER 4

THE INTERSECTION OF FOOD AND TECHNOLOGY

———

This past fall, in an interview with a company in the restaurant industry, my interviewer asked me, "What makes you tick?" The question caught me off guard. I managed to concoct some semblance of an answer, but in the days that followed, I couldn't stop thinking, *What would I have said if I had had more time to think?*

Upon reflection, I realized that it breaks down into two very simple things: people and food. What drives me on a day-to-day basis? The people in my life. They come in many forms. I am motivated in part by my interactions with strangers as I stand at the register of Saxbys for a few hours a couple of times a week. Even those minute-long interactions make me happy and give me energy. I'm particularly lucky in that sense because half of our customers are my peers, so the chances of friends walking through the door are pretty high.

The second aspect of "people" are those who I hold particularly near and dear to my heart: my parents, my closest friends, and the people who have watched me grow up. Being raised on a boarding school campus has given me a tight-knit community to call home. These people are my base, and as I've gotten older I've been fortunate enough to grow that base, adding people from Georgetown, from France, and from my summers working on Nantucket. The time I get to spend with those who know me best isn't always frequent, but it's always special. Whether my time with people is with strangers or close friends, I have always enjoyed making people happy.

One of the easiest ways to do that, I've learned, is through food. For many Saxbys customers, their trip to the coffee shop is a small high point of their day. It's a break, or a treat, or an energy booster. Regardless of the role it plays in their day, people tend to leave coffee shops happier than when they came in.

On a more personal level, food plays a central role in so many of my most important relationships. What does my family do when we all get together? We eat! What do I do with my friends for fun? We brunch! We try new restaurants or new bars, we grab coffee to catch up, we cook together at someone's house, we meet up at farmers' markets, and we even travel to local food events that are happening around Washington, DC.

Food is central to the lives of everyone. It offers us time to relax, to enjoy each other's company, and to indulge in different tastes and flavors. Sitting down to a meal together has suddenly become one of the only times of the day that our phone isn't attached to our hand. It allows us to stimulate senses we ignore the longer we spend staring at a computer screen.

Eve Turow Paul claims that the millennial obsession with food stems, at least in part, from the lack of social and sensory interaction we get in the rest of our lives, which we spend sitting at desks and staring at screens. In *A Taste of Generation Yum*, she elaborates on a conversation she had with Ken Friedman, the owner of multiple hot-spot restaurants in New York, including The Spotted Pig, which was designed specifically to encourage a sense of community.

Ken tells Eve the story of the time he overheard a customer say, "I've made more friends at The Spotted Pig than all throughout high school and college combined." It was music to Ken's ears because that was exactly the type of atmosphere he wanted to create. "He has, in fact, created the antithesis to the office cubicle: no borders, boundaries, screens, or headphones. What you get is real people, real food, real noise and intoxicating smells," Eve explains.

I knew she was right. There is something appealing about going out to a restaurant and being surrounded by people, noise, and good food. My friends and I love to go out and enjoy a carefree night full of exciting new drinks and dishes at one of DC's new restaurants. It is the one time of the day that everyone seems to silently agree on ignoring their phones for a couple of hours.

On the other hand, I have also watched the number of food deliveries among my generation skyrocket. I wanted to know: were people really going out to eat this much or was the explosion of food delivery apps like Uber Eats, Postmates, and Caviar encouraging people to stay in? How was technology, which had so seamlessly infiltrated into our everyday lives, influencing the food industry?

Christopher Myers, the same seasoned restaurateur mentioned in chapter 1, certainly had two cents to contribute. He was quick to tell me that one trend he's not so thrilled about as a restaurant manager is the trend toward food delivery. For one, he says, very few foods improve with time so the quality of the food that is being delivered is inferior to the quality of the food you'd get in a restaurant. Second, he says, "I like food. I love people. I like food. I love hospitality. It's hard to be hospitable when you're delivering a package to somebody."

Christopher views it as a form of lost business, not in the way that they are capturing less money, but that their relationship with customers is no longer the same. His reservations about the increase in food delivery services transfer into his opinion on the rise of social media as well. He can admit that social media is great; there has never before been an opportunity to get behind the scenes to hear what Anthony Bourdain has to say about food and wine.

Social media has the power to give you a passage into everyone else's world. However, it can also be taken to extremes, and that is where he sees it negatively impacting the quality human interaction. "When it comes to people walking down the street with their heads in their phones, even if they're being amused, people are no longer sharing the world in the same way."

He speaks to many fears about the millennial generation. Young people are now staying home in their living rooms rather than going to restaurants and being social. Whatever happened to going out for a meal by yourself, sitting at the bar, meeting a stranger, and having a conversation with someone you've never met? In Myers' opinion, technology is driving a wedge into our natural tendencies to be sociable, communal, and communicative. He would so much rather interact with his customers face to face and serve them in his own environment, showing a level of hospitality and appreciation that you can't show if you're just sending food to someone in a box. But, he admits about the rise in food to-go, "It's a thing. It's not going away because I think it's unfortunate."

On the other hand, Brett Schulman, the CEO of the fast-casual chain Cava, had a different take on technology's disruption of the food industry, and it was not the negative perception I expected. Instead, he emphasized how technology was revolutionizing the customer experience. If technology is used correctly and goes through the lens of "what customer problem is this solving," it can be great. If a customer asks for two scoops of harissa every time he/she walks into Cava, Cava now has the capability of recognizing that, expecting it, and using that information to connect with the customer outside the store by sending them harissa recipes via email. Because of the new versions of Point of Sale (POS) systems and other software infrastructure, companies can now collect and analyze all the raw data from customer transactions and use it to personalize the customer experience. That data analysis gives companies the power to gain insights on guest experience, typical length of stay in the store, creating an optimal store layout, and making informed real estate decisions.

The newest trend that is transforming retail in general—but that is certainly impacting the food industry—is a company's ability to meet customers wherever they are, physically, emotionally, and psycho-socially. "Brands no longer shout at their customers; it's a two-way conversation," Schulman explained. Restaurants, fast-casuals, and packaged goods companies are all being forced to reach a new level of engagement with their guests in order to create brand loyalty and a company-customer relationship that exists outside the transaction, primarily through social media interaction. That relationship is crucial because consumers are now bombarded with endless choices, and brand affinity is becoming the key to operating a sustainable business. The goal is no longer to simply get customers through the door; it's to inspire them to come back time and time again.

Todd Klein, a partner at Revolution Growth—a venture capital firm based in Washington, DC—explained that getting people to identify with your brand grants you good will with the customer, the ability to make a mistake and apologize for it. It also allows you more pricing flexibility because people understand the extra value you are providing and are willing to pay correspondingly.

The more trust customers place in a company, the more capable it is of withstanding a recession and achieving long-term success. That's where technology comes in. Companies must integrate new technologies that help them connect with their customers to build relationships in order to stay competitive. Because updated software has given restaurants the power to customize the customer experience, personalization has become the new expectation. A one-size-fits-all approach to marketing, sales, product development etc. is no longer successful. The brand has to support the customer's lifestyle.

One of the recurring themes throughout my conversations with people in the food industry—in food manufacturing, food market research, and restaurants—was this dilemma of how to market to and serve people who are inherently complex. I may be craving a kale salad one day, and then a DQ Blizzard the next. Vegans might be raving about their "clean eating" and environmentally friendly diet but still consuming a bag of Lays potato chips a day.

What we think we eat, or what we aspire to eat, is often vastly different than what we actually put into our bodies. This was proven by the previously mentioned study, in which Datassential conducted a survey asking people about their typical daily diet and what it consisted of. The results were high amounts of fruits and vegetables with little to no snacks. In the second survey, where they asked participants to keep a food diary for a week, the results were vastly different. People were snacking much more frequently than they admitted to in the first survey and eating fewer fruits and vegetables.

So how do you market to consumers who can so often be irrational or unpredictable? "It's more art than science," Dave Stever explained. Everything Ben & Jerry's puts out is consumer-tested and has passed a high benchmark. Everything *should* work. It costs $1.5 million to get a pint distributed on grocery store shelves nationwide. That isn't an investment they make without significant testing and positive indications that the product will sell. But the reality of the marketplace isn't always predictable and while some people may love certain items, those products might never make it to the masses.

Flavors will succeed in scoop shops but not in packaged lines because people shop differently in a grocery store than they do in a scoop shop. Ben & Jerry's has a unique way of celebrating their flavor failures. The factory in South Burlington, Vermont, is home to a flavor graveyard, in which each failed flavor gets a grave and customers are invited to walk through and observe past ideas. For Dave, the flavor graveyard reinforces the "art" or creative side of marketing because it reminds everybody to take risks rather than get too hung up on big data.

That being said, Stever, along with Brett Schulman of Cava and Mike Kostyo from Datassential, believe that big data, or gathering and analyzing huge amounts of information—particularly about your customers—is the ultimate marketing strategy of the future. Although Ben & Jerry's has an Instagram account, Instagram's logarithms decrease the level of control consumer packaged goods manufacturers have over their followers, views, and customer interaction. Facebook, on the other hand, has evolved into a major media and advertising channel. The newest challenge is how to gather the consumer's data and not be at the mercy of Facebook to reach them. "It's really about getting data, owning the data, and getting into the consumer's day-to-day life at the right time through the right messaging. The only way you're going to do that is through acquiring the data through all the different apps and your own websites," Stever explains.

While we may witness a technology backlash as millennials ditch their phones to enjoy a night of good food and conversation, begin to reconsider traditional industries like agriculture, and cook more in their own homes, it is equally clear that technology isn't going anywhere. The global market for food delivery is valued at around 83 billion euros, which is approximately 102 billion dollars and equates to 1 percent of the total food market and 4 percent of food sold in restaurants and fast-food chains. The industry is expected to grow at 3.5 percent for the next five years.

More and more people are latching on to the new trend as they realize they can receive restaurant-quality food in their own home within a matter of minutes. And from a company rather than a consumer perspective, technology is now everything. Tracking data on customers no longer just gives a leg up in marketing. It's now the basic technique. Social media channels are the new modes of communication between companies and customers, and even within agriculture, technology is bringing new levels of sustainability and efficient production methods.

Mike Kostyo of Datassential explained, "You can't just ignore it now. In the past we've focused on either restaurant or manufacturing technology, but now this technology is really affecting agriculture and how we grow and harvest food." It sounds to me like technology, in the hands of millennials, has the potential to revolutionize the food industry for the better.

CHAPTER 5

SOCIAL MEDIA: A POWERFUL VOICE

In this day and age, it feels impossible to talk about technology without talking about social media too. One thing that popped up over and over, particularly in my conversations with small food business owners, was the shift from traditional marketing channels to social media. Vanessa, cofounder of Health-Ade Kombucha, and Chloe, the owner of Chloe's Pops, both spoke to the importance of honesty in customer relations in their marketing strategy as well.

Chloe explained that her customer interactions and conversations now occur via social media channels. Commenting and messaging on Instagram have become the main way in which she gauges her company's product quality and customer satisfaction. One of her most successful initiatives was her blog, Brain Freeze, which, in Chloe's words, "offers parents advice on how to answer their kids' food questions with *some* degree of grace and humor."

The blog stemmed from Chloe's realization that her company was a reflection of her values as a parent. "Wouldn't it be so fun to have a place where moms, dads, and caregivers who experience the highs, lows, and in-betweens of parenting come together and vent?" Chloe writes in her initial post on Brain Freeze. The publication has allowed her to create an online community where her customers can come together, not just as fruit pop consumers, but as parents who deal with their kids every single day and have stories to share—stories that will make you want to laugh, cry, and everything in between.

Vanessa, too, emphasized the growing importance of social media, saying, "There's a momentum in social media that hasn't existed before. It's vital to edge your way into that community." But for Health-Ade, digital technology offers another exciting aspect in addition to social media—online education. As soon as they learned of the astronomically high number of Google searches related to Kombucha each day, Health-Ade immediately made it their priority to become the leading, educational voice on what Kombucha is so that they can reach farther than customers to people who are just curious about kombucha in general. They devote an entire page of their website to "What is Kombucha?" as they walk the visitor through the definition, the ingredients, and the fermentation process. The last page, of course, explains just what makes their kombucha the best.

As I wondered whether Chloe and Vanessa's stories were isolated incidents, I happened upon a *Forbes* article titled "Why Word of Mouth Marketing Is the Most Important Social Media." The article stated that 92 percent of consumers believe recommendations from friends and family over all other forms of advertising and 64 percent of marketing executives believe that word of mouth is the most effective form of marketing. So why have leaders in the marketing industry still not mastered it?

"The problem is that for the last few years, marketers have been focused on 'collecting' instead of 'connecting,'" explains Kimberly Whitler, author of the *Forbes* article. The 4Ps—Product, Place, Promotion, and Price—have long been the foundation of marketing. But Kimberly urges a new focus, the 3Es—Engage, Equip, and Empower—given the digital age. Even the largest companies are making efforts to engage with individual customers online.

Nike support is known for responding to customer tweets within a matter of minutes. My Starbucks Idea offers a medium for customers to propose new ideas so the company understands what its customers are looking for and customers feel that their voices are being heard. Morton's Steakhouse even delivered a bag of steak, shrimp, and potatoes to a customer who had jokingly requested they meet him at the airport with his order via Twitter.

These initiatives don't go unnoticed, and they certainly build credibility. The second "E," equip, refers to giving your customers something to talk about. Whether it's kombucha quality that's second to none or relatable stories of parenting that have customers interacting with each other through your blog, your brand should find a way to stay relevant in the lives of your customers, often by simply understanding them.

The last component, "empower," addresses the question of how. Give your customers a platform—whether that's Instagram, Twitter, Facebook, an app, or a website—on which they can reach you. The onus then lies on the company to listen and respond because the whole idea is that the company-consumer relationship is now a two-way street. "Jerry [*of Ben & Jerry's*] once said that the strongest bond you can build with your customers is over shared values," Dave Stever told me. From where I'm sitting, Jerry was way ahead of his time.

Perhaps even more powerful than a brand's social media presence is what its customers are saying about it via their own social media accounts. Rachel Hosie writes for the UK-based newspaper *The Independent.* As she sat down to brunch with her mother one day, she immediately pulled out her phone to snap some pictures. Her mother, evidently embarrassed, suggested that they explain to the servers that Rosie was a journalist. "But it was nothing to do with me being a journalist. I'm just a millennial," Rosie writes.

Millennials aren't just snapping photos to document what they eat, but also to decide where to eat. Just the other night, three friends and I spent at least five minutes trolling a restaurant's Instagram before we decided which item to order off the menu. As I was searching for just the right brunch venue for my mom and me, I made sure to scroll the Instagram photos from each restaurant before making a reservation. And whenever I see a particularly mouthwatering photo on Instagram, I tap the picture to find out where it's from so I can add the restaurant to my constantly growing list of new places to try.

Being able to see a picture of a restaurant's menu items has always been a major factor in determining what we order. The same phenomenon explains why cookbooks are filled with photos of the products of its recipes. With the rise of Instagram, we now have those photos available to us even before we decide where to eat so a restaurant's Instagram presence is becoming a major component of its ability to attract customers.

Restaurants are learning to produce aesthetically pleasing food because, beyond their own Instagram presence, they cannot control the photos posted of their food. Customers will add geotags and hashtags that link the restaurant to the photos they post of their food, so the prettier food is, the more attention you'll receive. "Social media is *the* tool for finding new places to eat," confirms Justin Schuble, the highly coveted photographer and Instagram influencer, @dcfoodporn.

With the ever-increasing presence of food photos on Instagram, those who call themselves "influencers" are gaining popularity and power within the food scene. *Bon Appétit*'s Michelle Ruiz defines an influencer as "the much-used, vaguely icky term for social media wunderkinds parlaying their fabulous feeds into new media empires in fashion, art, and increasingly, food," a title I couldn't help but love.

I was taken aback the first time I heard the word "influencer." I wasn't even aware that all the food accounts and health gurus I followed on Instagram had a name, but the more I thought about it, the more accurate I realized it was. These "influencers" who often have upward of 500,000 followers on Instagram are quite literally influencing where we choose to eat.

A great example is the acclaimed Black Tap Burger & Shake in New York City, whose proliferation of photos on Instagram led to hours-long lines at their locations, an entire story on Buzzfeed, and a feature on ABC's *The Chew*. I was lucky enough to speak with Emily Morse, one of the young women behind @new_fork_city, one of Instagram's top-rated food accounts, with over 887,000 followers, and she told me the story of the moment she realized just how much influence she had on Instagram. The first summer after @new_fork_city had started, Emily was working in The Hamptons. Her friend had recommended a bake shop that sold these amazing cinnamon rolls, so Emily tried one and immediately posted a photo of one of the rolls on @new_fork_city. The next day she went back with her mom to grab some cinnamon rolls to bring back to the family, and the bake shop had sold out of the cinnamon rolls within an hour of opening.

The employees of the small bake shop said they'd had a really strange rush of customers that morning. "We realized," Emily said, "that it was probably because we had posted a picture the day before." It was a big moment for the girls of @new_fork_city, realizing they had the power to influence not only their followers, but also the success of the bakery.

Having heard Emily's perspective, I set out to speak with another foodie influencer, one closer to home. Brittany Arnett is the young woman behind the primarily DC-based Instagram handle, @toastedtable, who launched her account a few years after @new_fork_city. @toastedtable took off quickly, with her first photo of avocado toast gaining over 1,000 likes on Instagram. Two years later, Brittany's Instagram handle has roughly 6,000 followers, but one of the struggles she has faced is learning how to evolve with Instagram.

The growth of @toastedtable has stagnated since Instagram changed its logarithm. It's more difficult now to attract new followers or get as many likes. Her goal is eventually to make it to 10,000 followers, at which point Instagram considers you a "valued user" and your growth skyrockets. Once you've hit 10,000, it becomes easier and easier to gain new followers. The social media learning curve was steep and full of nuances. By now, Brittany has developed her own toolkit of strategies. She uses hash-tags very deliberately, by posting a bunch on her photos and then hiding them from the comments section so that her followers don't necessarily see all of them.

She also does her best to tag other well-known handles in her photos to gain more traction. And every time she posts a photo, she immediately looks through all the other posts under the same hashtag or location, and likes and comments on hundreds of them. "I literally just sit there and tap non-stop," she explains. "Liking and commenting on other peoples' photos fuels more likes and comments on your own content and attracts more followers." It's those not-so-subtle unspoken rules of social media: like for like, follow for follow, or comment for comment, that have all come to dominate the game of Instagram influencers. If you can get someone to click on your name from your comment and they like your content, chances are they'll follow you.

Brittany also explained that there are two different types of food Instagrams—those that only post original content, i.e., photos and food that they have created or photographed, and "repost accounts" that take photos from other Instagrams and repost them on their own page, giving photo credit in the comments section. Repost accounts tend to do better than originals because they can search for the highest quality photo out there and post it, whereas it's much more difficult for one person to get the best content and the best photo every single time. She made it clear to me that success on social media stems from your strategy as much as the quality of your posts.

Virtual relationships have become increasingly important to the food blogger community. Brittany highlighted the sharing culture within the food Instagram community. She and @ dcfoodporn will exchange ideas, feedback, and new places to try, or she'll reach out to @captaintruffle for great restaurant recommendations in DC. Some of the most famous food bloggers tend to do things in groups. They'll attend restaurant openings and other food-related events together, often because they are so prominent that restaurants will invite them for the free publicity they receive in return. That allows these bloggers to meet up in person and collaborate on content. They all have to have achieved a certain status on Instagram before companies are allowed to pay them to photograph their food. With 5,000 followers, Brittany gets offered free food or discounts at certain restaurants if she comes to take photos. For anyone with upward of 10,000 followers, places will pay to have them come take photos of the restaurant's dishes and then offer free food on top of that.

"Restaurants and bars are increasingly giving influencers a seat at the industry table, reaching out to them alongside critics and traditional media," Michelle Ruiz writes in her *Bon Appétit* article. While there may be some reluctance among the restaurant industry to give these sometimes shockingly young masters of social media free meals and sometimes even free buffets of the entire menu, it can often pay off for a restaurant to be featured on that world-famous Instagram. "You really need that influencer crowd to come in," says Emily Dickens, the director of sales and events at 50 Eggs, a culinary and hospitality firm located in Miami and Las Vegas.

If there's one thing I took away from my discussions with these hip, young foodie influencers, it's that their relationships with restaurants are symbiotic. There's a give and take on both sides, and as soon as the balance is tipped in favor of one, it doesn't take long for drama to ensue. @dcfoodporn and @new_fork_city, two top 'grams, both expressed frustration with being taken advantage of by companies and restaurants due to their young age. On the flip side, restaurants aren't thrilled with the occasional influencers who have let their number of followers go to their heads and suddenly demand free four-course meals, not only for themselves, but for any number of friends they decide to bring along as well.

"There's no rule book for how to make a career out of being an influencer, or an Instagram star, or whatever you want to call it," Justin affirms, but as the number of food-based Instagram accounts continues to skyrocket, only the best and brightest will reach Instagram-verified stardom. Whether or not these social media savvy photographers achieve fame, they are all inevitably taking part in a movement that gives power back to consumers.

By communicating among ourselves, we are forcing restaurants to comply with our high standards of food across a variety of factors—be it presentation, health, customizability, or photo-ability. Millennials are using social media to help dictate food trends, create food hot spots, and credit those restaurants, cafes, or bakeries that we deem deserving of our attention. Social media has given us a powerful voice.

CHAPTER 6

OUR FOOD GURUS: THE PEOPLE WE LISTEN TO, KNOW, AND TRUST

—

Our knowledge of food and health, like almost everything these days, seems to be moving from traditional sources like doctors, medical journals, or the Health section of newspapers to social media. "We don't have a lot of evidence-based research or studies, so we're working off of perception, ability to influence people, and what contributes to health," explains Carol Day, a certified nutritionist at Georgetown University.

Gone are the days of seeking nutrition advice from your general care physician and relying on the incorporation of each of the food groups into your diet. In fact, I rarely hear anyone talking about the food pyramid anymore. Today, it's all about the latest sugar alternative, the newest superfood, or the most recent dietary supplement. Instagram plays a huge part in that and so do the dieticians, food bloggers, health nuts, and self-proclaimed foodies who use social media as their primary form of engagement with their clients and followers.

Melissa Hartwig is one of the greatest examples of someone who started out on a personal journey to redefine her relationship with food in a healthier way and ended up a celebrity in the world of nutrition. In less than a decade, she transitioned from a young woman who had spent the past few years of her life with a severe drug abuse problem to the creator of the Whole30 program and the author of two best-selling books. She can't even explain how. "Weirdly, in my eyes, people started following my blog. Maybe it was because I dropped F-bombs all the time. Maybe it was because I wasn't afraid to tell it like it was. My writing was pretty candid but also pretty humorous." The Whole30 program involves eliminating certain food groups, like legumes, dairy, sugar, and grains, from your diet for thirty days in order to re-evaluate how foods are affecting your body. Whole30 describes the eliminated foods as "the most common craving-inducing, blood sugar disrupting, gut-damaging, inflammatory" food groups and has found them to be the most commonly problematic across a broad range of people.

"If you had asked me before Whole30, I would have said I'm the healthiest person in the world," said Melissa in her interview with Jason Wachob, founder and CEO of the mindbodygreen Podcast. Once she had stopped using drugs, she started going to the gym too much, becoming an extreme bodybuilder and over-exercising. She had essentially replaced drugs with fitness. But once she and her Whole30 cofounder, Dallas, spent thirty days on a type of paleo diet as an experiment, her mindset shifted. She realized that her relationship with food was dysfunctional and that the extent to which she had been using food as punishment or reward was harmful.

She even compared her abuse of food to her abuse of drugs. "Feeling out of control, overconsuming, hating yourself for it, the guilt and the shame that comes with it. The isolation of the behavior . . . Am I talking about heroin or candy?" People could relate to her behavior. Once Melissa had posted it on her blog, hundreds of people chose to do the Whole30 program and reported similar experiences.

"When two people have a good experience, it's cool," says Melissa. "When a hundred people have a good experience and it's similar, you realize this is a thing." What began as an experiment between friends is now a program that's being lauded by doctors, trending on *The New York Times Bestsellers* list, and expanding to a community of millions of people. The newest food and nutrition trends are no longer coming from experts with medical degrees but from self-discovered and experimental health bloggers. They are now the first-movers, and the doctors stick around to evaluate the validity of the new trends.

In contrast to all of the health and wellness accounts that have flooded Instagram in recent years, there are equally as many purely food-based accounts. These often promote indulgence just as much as they do moderation. @new_fork_city is a special example of a food Instagram because it was one of the first. In the winter of 2014, Emily, Gillian, and Natalie launched @ new_fork_city, an account that posts mouthwatering photos of foods at hot spots all throughout New York City.

"It started before food Instagrams were a trend," Emily told me. "We kind of just realized we were posting too many food photos to our personal accounts," and thus, @new_fork_city was created out of pure necessity. The girls decided it was time to launch an Instagram account devoted entirely to pictures of food. Little did they know that three years later, they would have a following of 862,000 people and over 2,500 posts.

Within its first year, @new_fork_city received its first offer from a brand that was looking for a partnership. From there, things grew quickly and organically. More and more restaurants and food companies were reaching out to the girls to collaborate and create mutual relationships. When I asked

Emily about that transition, she told me, "I've had this little insight that I wouldn't have had otherwise—the legal aspect of it. We have to do contracts, we have lawyers, we had to trademark the name, all of that fun stuff."

Emily, Gillian, and Natalie have far more business and legal experience than your average twenty-one-year-olds. The only downside of all the buzz? "Because we are so young, in the past people have tried to take advantage of us," Emily admits. They have learned early to be wary of certain businesses and to define explicitly the way they expect to be treated by their partners.

Beyond overcoming legal and business complications, I wanted to know what Emily thought made @new_fork_city so successful. Why do so many people follow them? She mentioned a myriad of things that she thinks define @new_fork_city as a brand and separate it from the newly crowded web of food Instagrams and bloggers. One of them initially surprised me: "We definitely focus on comfort food. A lot of food Instagrams focus on healthy food or fitness, and while we do think that's important, we post a lot of foods with cheese or desserts and a lot of unhealthy foods," Emily said.

Capturing photos of the opposite end of the food spectrum— foods that are extravagant and unhealthy to the extreme—has clearly been a successful business model for @new_fork_city.

As eagerly as we millennials have launched ourselves into the health food craze, there's no question that we like to indulge too. If food Instagrams provide us with sources of inspiration for healthy meals, they encourage us equally successfully to splurge every once in a while.

Emily also emphasized the importance of quality over quantity for @new_fork_city. The girls hold high standards for the photo submissions they post: a sharp focus, optimal lighting, and a focus on the individual food item rather than a table spread are all trademarks of their photos. Upholding rigorous photo quality standards is crucial to their continuing success, as the girls are currently spread across the country at different universities and can't be in New York as much as they'd like. It is tradition, however, to cram as many different meals and photos into every trip back home so that they can stock up on good content.

Lastly, the three founders stick to their core values. "We'll never do a collaboration or partnership with a brand or restaurant that we wouldn't otherwise promote and suggest to our followers," Emily tells me. "We're young. We love to help businesses we love. Making money is great, but we also just love to support brands and businesses that we think are worthy."

Deliberate or not, it was a smart business decision, because it coincides directly with the larger cultural trend in food toward business transparency, shared values and authenticity between the company and consumer.

The next Instagram sensation I chatted with was Brittany Arnett, the creator behind @toastedtable, a food account based primarily on pictures of toast. I had to ask, "Why avocado toast? What makes it so special?" The first thing out of her mouth was its versatility. But behind her creative applications and renditions of the combination was a personal story. "When I was in high school, I was SUPER calorie-conscious. I thought bread was the enemy. Everything in my life was made without bread because I thought, *Bread is bad for you.*" It wasn't until her mom sat her down and they decided to confront the issue together that Brittany began to overcome her fear of bread.

Once she started looking at its nutritional value, she realized that bread, whole-wheat bread in particular, is healthy in moderate quantities because its complex carbs will keep you full for longer. Coincidentally, right around the time Brittany was re-introducing bread into her life, avocado toast started to become a trend. But avocado was just the beginning. "You can literally put anything on top of a piece of toast and make it a meal that will taste good," Brittany says. "There are certain ingredients that just taste better on bread." And if Brittany alone doesn't convince you, just try asking one of her roughly 6,000 Instagram followers.

Whereas @new_fork_city is a successful example of a "repost account," @toastedtable and @dcfoodporn both post original content. Unlike the other two, Justin Schuble has decided to pursue a full-blown career through his Instagram account, @dcfoodporn. "This is a full-time job, whether or not I treat it like that. In terms of time commitment and what people expect of me, it keeps me really busy. My goal was to figure out how to make enough money off of that to not have to work a 9-5 job," he explained.

So far, it seems to be going well. Justin is already "verified" by the blue check on Instagram, meaning that Instagram has confirmed that his account authentically represents him as a celebrity or public figure, and he just managed to break 200,000 followers this past December. He attributes his success to constantly talking to other Instagram influencers, learning from his mistakes, and getting as much feedback as he can from both his followers and the brands he works with.

Similarly to @new_fork_city, Justin faced a learning curve as his Instagram popularity grew. He learned the hard way that people occasionally try to take advantage of his time and his photos. He has since learned to get all contracts in writing as well as to negotiate for himself. One of his biggest learning moments, however, was a less serious incident.

The popsicle brand, Good Humor, had asked him to take

pictures of their products at the national monuments in DC. So naturally, he bought a pack of popsicles and headed out there. Once he'd made it to the monuments, he took the pack out. "Everything was melted, and I was getting attacked by bees. It was a total disaster, and I was freaking out!" Justin says, laughing now as he looks back. "It was a pretty good learning experience to know to plan for the worst-case scenario."

I was intrigued by the ins and outs of what probably sounds like a dream job to most people. How could there be any downsides to a job that pays you to eat and photograph food? But Justin made it clear that his job wasn't all sunshine and rainbows. "I have to live and breathe what I do, so I'm kind of always working and never working at the same time," he explains. He is forced to worry constantly about cultivating this perfect social media image and to keep his phone with him wherever he goes, which makes it difficult for him to be fully present with his friends and family.

That being said, it was clear that Justin loves what he does. There's a certain level of creativity required to find and post good photos as well as a certain analysis to finding the worthwhile food fads. Are they photogenic? Colorful? Customizable? Are they extreme like superfoods or extremely overindulgent? Are they unique, elevated, and exciting? These are all criteria Justin looks for before he decides to photograph.

His job certainly never gets boring. "The cool thing is I'll post about anything from a new donut shop to a $500 tasting menu in DC. There's a lot of variety in what I post and what people want to see." With the boom in millennial food culture and the explosion of food in social media, Justin's job isn't going anywhere soon.

What ties these seemingly unique four "food gurus" together is that they are like us: they're not perfect, they are subject to human error, and they don't claim to be geniuses or have a perfect diet. Melissa Hartwig began as a drug user, Brittany had an unhealthy relationship with bread, and Justin completely bombed one of his first assignments. They are human. They allow us to relate to them. And they, too, lie at the heart of the millennial food movement because they too, are reacting against big business and cliché, traditional health messages.

Each of them has learned to be wary of larger companies trying to take advantage of them or trying to steal their content. Melissa offers an aggressive approach that she created and lived by herself. She and her two million followers are proof of the success of the Whole30 program. @new_fork_city and @dcfoodporn are like friends who keep you updated on all of the newest, up-and-coming eateries in New York City and Washington, DC and who understand the need to indulge in your cravings. Brittany is a college student who has offered us healthy toast combinations which all involve eating actual bread, instead of forcing us to give up carbs as so many mainstream diets would lead us to do. Because we can relate to them, because we trust and recognize them, these social media masters are the people we look to and listen to for the latest trends.

CHAPTER 7

THE INSPIRATION: ENTREPRENEURS IN FOOD

———

As I tried to reconcile all I had heard, read, and seen regarding some of the millennial trends that were shaping the food industry, one group of people stood out to me as a beacon of hope for the millennial generation. These were the food entrepreneurs. In every single one of my conversations with people who had started their own food businesses, I was inspired.

I became more and more sure that with people like them leading the pack, our generation was moving the food industry in the right direction. They treated their products and their customers with the utmost care, revolutionizing the company-customer relationship, upping the standards of food and service quality, and staying true to their core values. Speaking with them was by far the most fun part of my research, and I feel compelled to share their stories with you.

PINEAPPLE IN DC: VANESSA, NEKISIA, CHLOE, AND ANITA

This fall, I had the chance to attend a panel on female entrepreneurship in the food industry, sponsored by Pineapple DC, a collaborative of over 10,000 people who meet off and online to bring women together around good food. As informative as Pineapple DC's event "Women in Food Deliver" was, it was honestly more fun than anything else. Here were four fabulous young women, each of whose jobs I would jump at, who had come to DC not to compete with each other or aggressively push their own brand, but to collaborate and share their experiences.

Nekisia had started her own granola company, Anita owned her own non-dairy, coconut yogurt company, Chloe had launched a line of all-natural popsicles made from only real fruit and a touch of cane sugar, and Vanessa was the cofounder of a leading premium kombucha brand, Health-Ade. Who were they speaking to? A hodgepodge group of women whose only commonality was some form of passion for the food industry.

I found myself surrounded by Georgetown graduate students, a young woman who was in the process of launching her own new product, a woman who worked for Ashbury Labeling, a firm that mediates between the FDA and numerous food companies to create accurate nutritional labels, and a food blogger/Instagram influencer. I wanted to meet everyone. I wanted to hear each of their stories. I wanted to be friends with all of them. Part of me was in shock that these high-achieving, inspirational women who were years ahead of me in their careers were so accessible, friendly, and easy to chat with, but the other part of me felt right at home. These women represent the reasons I want to break into the food industry. They are creative, they are collaborative, they are risk-takers, and they, too, are driven by people and food.

While each of the four CEO/Founders on the panel had a unique story, a few shared learning experiences among all four of them resonated with me. One was their level of innovation and gumption. They all agreed on the lack of clear guidance or direction that exists for starting a food company. "There's certainly no handbook" was the general consensus.

Nekisia Davis, the founder of Early Bird Granola, even admitted that she hadn't meant to start a company, but that somehow she accidentally had, and it all began with a Google search: "How do you make granola?" Her original recipe is still her best-selling granola to this day.

Chloe from Chloe's Fruit had a similar story. She had never intended to sell popsicles or even to create a packaged product that would be sold in supermarkets, but when she froze her leftover yogurt from her frozen yogurt shop and distributed it to her friends and employees as popsicles, she discovered a market for it. Those popsicles became her product and the reason behind her success.

Each of the founders had begun creating their products in the small, humble confines of their personal kitchens: crafting Kombucha in a friend's closet, filling the fridge she shared with her boyfriend entirely with five gallons of coconut yogurt, or throwing various combinations of water, fruit, and cane sugar into a blender until she found the best one. Not one of them knew where their product was going to take them.

They described the various pivot points of their companies, the growing pains, and the constant feeling of fumbling along as you go. Nekisia said if there was one thing she wished she had known before starting, it was how hard it was going to be. Yet among their stories of hardships, roadblocks, and failures, the most resounding piece of advice was "Just do it." They advised us all not to let the idea of perfect get in the way of "great." If you can create a product that's sellable, you're halfway there.

Second, they all agreed that people management had been the biggest challenge of growing their business. Having experienced business relationships that went awry, they emphasized the importance of hiring people who truly "get it" and will do everything in their power to uphold the expected standard of quality.

Vanessa spoke in particular about the difficult transition from the responsibility lying solely on her, Daina, and Justin to hiring more people to carry some of that responsibility and brand representation. "The dependency shifts from you to a dependency on many. It's both the challenge and the reward," Vanessa explained. It was difficult for them to hire the right people in order to expand and represent the exact culture the three founders had created as well as to take the company to the next level.

The four business owners also offered a similar attitude toward partnerships, emphasizing that partner companies should share your values and demonstrate that they care about your mission and your brand specifically. Nekisia, Vanessa, Chloe, and Anita emphasized the importance of an alignment of values throughout the panel. In addition to behind-the-scenes relationships between employees and retail partners, shared values were the main form of communication and interaction with their customers.

Nekisia mentioned that during her time in the restaurant industry, she had felt dispensable as a human being until she worked for Danny Myers at Gramercy Tavern in New York. "He was the first boss who cared more about the people working for him than the restaurant's bottom line," she explained, a quality she has worked hard to translate into her own company.

When I asked her about the rising trends in health awareness and company ethics, Nekisia said that the restaurant industry is already being affected. These trends have changed the landscape of food in New York City because people no longer go to restaurants now unless they know where the food is sourced from. Transparency in every aspect of your business is the new key to success. The idea of honesty and transparency vis-à-vis her customers is truly the baseline of Early Bird Granola. Nekisia prides her company on customer experience. Above everything else, each bag of granola she sells is about how she makes her customers feel through that interaction.

The slogan of Vanessa's kombucha company, Health-Ade is "Follow your gut!" This not only represents Vanessa's mindset but also the entrepreneurial spirit of the millennial generation. Their slogan originated from its double-entendre. Kombucha is rich in probiotics, good bacteria, and healthy acids, so it's good for your gut, but "Follow your gut!" also represents the trust you need to have in yourself. Health-Ade encourages its consumers to follow their gut, not just to the probiotics in kombucha but also to their inner purpose. Vanessa hopes their slogan will allow both brand and individual consumer expression through the purchase of Health-Ade. Her ability to know, understand, and connect with Health-Ade consumers will dictate the company's future success and longevity. "Consumers aren't just interested in better for you, they're interested in what's real and what's good for you," Vanessa explained, and that is what Health-Ade works to provide.

TWO MEN FROM UNION KITCHEN: CULLEN GILCHRIST AND ANDY BROWN

I also had the chance to listen and speak with some of the food entrepreneurs who were central to the urban culture of our nation's capital. At the heart of food entrepreneurship in Washington, DC, is Union Kitchen, the food accelerator started by Cullen Gilchrist and Jonas Singer. Since its founding in 2013 as the first commercial kitchen and incubator in DC, it has seen over 120 businesses come through, including Swizzler, the famous gourmet hot dog truck, JRINK, the DC-wide juice brand, and District Doughnut, one of DC's renowned donut shops. When asked in an interview with Georgetown University Eating Society what led him to create Union Kitchen, Cullen said, "It was the idea that by creating Union Kitchen, we could create a more interesting place to live." He thought DC was lacking a strong food scene. Because so much of culture is based on food, Cullen believes that by founding Union Kitchen, he has made DC a better city.

Union Kitchen's goal is to build successful food businesses and to provide an environment in which food businesses can be successful. Union Kitchen owns everything from delivery trucks and a 3,700-square-foot commercial kitchen to a warehouse and several grocery stores. A large part of their mission is to create a local footprint and to give food entrepreneurs an environment that allows them to grow regionally and nationally.

After speaking with food entrepreneurs like Shizu Okusa from JRINK, Andy Brown from Eat Pizza, and Samy K from Snacklins, whose successes began at Union Kitchen, I was curious to hear Cullen's side of the story. What made these business owners so successful in their endeavors? What did Union Kitchen look for when it selected the businesses to accommodate? Cullen listed all the traits you might expect— someone who is smart, who is going to hustle, who is going to work hard—but most importantly, someone who has the ability to learn and be coached by others.

He also mentioned that while starting a food business requires a certain level of commitment and a solid belief in your idea, you have to remember that it's not about you. It's ultimately about the customers who are looking for a solution. To sell a product, you have to solve a problem. Cullen said he has many people who come through with ideas they don't see on grocery store shelves. "There's a reason they don't see them.

People usually don't want them." You have to make a product people want that is also scalable.

Cullen's ultimate piece of advice for people looking to start a food business is to become an expert at what you do. "If you're not great at what you do, you're probably replaceable," he readily admitted. If you can gain expertise in your area, you can tell a story that connects to consumers, which will better sell the product. At the end of the day, the founder who created the product and who believes wholeheartedly in the product will drive the company forward. If the passion is there, the next step is expertise. Then, you might just have something.

Andy Brown joined the accelerator program at Union Kitchen this past January. He is the founder of Eat Pizza, a company that sells "frozen pizza that actually tastes like pizza." The pizza also happens to be organic, natural, and GMO-free. He is currently in talks to grow regionally with Whole Foods, with the goal of having his pizza in stores from south Virginia all the way to Connecticut. His next big project is building his own Eat Pizza factory in Rockville, Virginia.

Andy's story, like those of many of the food entrepreneurs I've spoken with, was not a typical one. He started as a DJ at The Tombs, a popular student bar just off Georgetown University's campus. He then worked at Mission, a restaurant in DC, where he became a general manager and continued on to open Hawthorne with them. He spent over a year and a half there before he decided he wanted to open his own pizza place.

When he met with Cullen Gilchrist, cofounder and owner of Union Kitchen, Cullen recommended that Andy sell frozen pizza. "I remember thinking that's a terrible idea—end of meeting," Andy says. But the more he thought about it, he realized the magic of selling a packaged good. It allows for much greater scalability than opening a restaurant. Andy now has the opportunity to build a facility in Rockville and distribute his product all the way across the country to California.

Andy acknowledges there have been plenty of challenges in this endeavor. Getting stores to distribute his product has been one of his biggest struggles so far. The stores don't want to sell your product because you don't have the distribution network, but distributors don't want you because you don't have the sales. It becomes a game of playing them against each other until someone finally caves.

He still faces these problems today. His main advice is "Hire yourself out of a job." It may sound counterintuitive, but if you have the idea in your head that no one else can do what you do, your business will never grow. He advised business owners to do whatever they are strong at, and farm out everything else. In order to grow, you have to relinquish absolute control over every aspect of the process. That can be hard—to let things go out of your hands and to trust other people—but in order to develop a business, it's absolutely necessary.

FROM FINANCE TO FOOD: SHIZU OKUSA AND BRETT SCHULMAN

Shizu Okusa, the founder of JRINK juicery in DC, and Brett Schulman, the CEO of Cava, both began their careers in finance. Brett described his previous career on Wall Street as a case of the "Sunday night blues." Every Monday morning, he wanted to hit snooze and find something he was passionate about. His first venture into the food industry was the launch of a natural snack food company with his wife. His family had always been into healthy eating and conscious of what they put into their bodies. They knew it didn't have to be difficult to eat better, so they launched a line of healthy snack bars.

That was just the beginning. In 2009, Brett was introduced to the partners at Cava Mezze restaurant. At the time, they only owned one full-service restaurant and had begun to sell some of their dips in Whole Foods. Brett and the partners hit it off immediately. By 2011, they had opened their first "chef casual" restaurant, and today, they currently operate thirty-five Cava locations and five full-service Cava Mezze restaurants.

Shizu Okusa had previously worked at Goldman Sachs and was working in finance at the World Bank when she began juicing on the side. At the time, there were no food delivery apps. "It was so hard to stay healthy when we were so busy. What's a quick way to do that?" she was asking herself, just as she started to bring juices in from home. She quickly realized how convenient juice was for her, as well as the market opportunity that existed in DC, where there were really no juice companies at the time.

"It all happened really organically, I would say," Shizu added, no pun intended! Once they discovered Union Kitchen, they moved into its commercial kitchen to try to launch their juice business on a large scale. Today, they operate five juice locations in DC and offer both instantaneous and pre-scheduled deliveries.

Shizu spoke with pride about her company's success, but she also acknowledged the fact that things get more complicated as the company gets bigger. "I miss and remember with a lot of gratitude the early days . . . We were juicing ourselves and spilling cucumber pulp everywhere. I used to wear garbage bags over my shoes when we delivered in the snow, because I couldn't afford boots!" she said, laughing. JRINK has come a long way since their days in Union Kitchen.

As we chatted further, Shizu also spoke to the same challenges that previous entrepreneurs had mentioned. As a small company who can't offer the same salaries of places like sweetgreen and Cava, it's not always easy to hire and retain the right people, nor is it easy to find "good" money. "You don't want to give business away to the wrong people," Shizu said. She found it difficult to find people she could trust, whether that was potential employees or investors.

I also noticed that Shizu placed a similar emphasis on JRINK's company-customer relationship as Vanessa did with Health-Ade and Nekisia did with Early Bird Granola. She aims to treat every customer like a real person and to engage in conversation with each one who walks through their doors, striving to offer both excellent customer service and an excellent product. "We *have* to be an experience," she told me, acknowledging that if people are going to spend $9 or $10 on a juice, it has to be worth it.

JRINK uses social media avidly to connect with their consumers. Shizu described it as a way to talk to consumers anywhere, anytime. It allows JRINK to stay on top of quality control and also to communicate directly with consumers to get their feedback. Here was yet another small, local business that prioritized its understanding of and relationship with its consumers in order to set itself apart from the competition.

MY IDOL: MILLENNIAL FOOD
CONSULT, EVE TUROW PAUL

Last but not least, one of the most fascinating entrepreneurs I had the chance to speak with was Eve Turow Paul, the only millennial food consultant I am aware of to this day. Eve graduated from Amherst College in 2009 with a degree in psychology and was planning to continue on to get her PhD. But after one summer of working in a lab, she changed her mind. It wasn't the experiments that she loved, but the opportunity to gather all the research and tell a story with it.

Unfortunately, she happened to graduate smack dab in the middle of the economic recession, so after struggling to find a job, she moved to Argentina to live on the peso and write for an expat newspaper that allowed her to review a cooking class and a food service. "It was really the first time I realized that food was this amazing combination of economics, politics, agriculture, and religion and all of these different things," she explained to me excitedly.

After just three months in Argentina, she managed to get hired back in the states at the Communications department of the Economic Policy Institute (EPI). Simultaneously, she pitched NPR to write about food and began working on "Kitchen Window," a food column on recipe development and food history. But it wasn't until her return to school for her master's degree that she realized she and all her peers were spending the entirety of their discretionary income on food.

In college, she reflected, she hadn't cared about what she ate at all. In fact, she would routinely lose weight upon her returns to campus and sometimes, she didn't even care enough to remember to eat all the time. "I would like microwave a bowl of rice with some weird shredded cheese on top and that was my meal. Or several dinners of captain crunch," she admitted, laughing. But all of a sudden, during grad school in New York, she was saving up to go to an expensive, underground dinner or showing her friends pictures of the food she had made.

Her background at the EPI, which had given her a strong understanding of how badly the economic recession was going to impact our generation, only deepened her confusion. She couldn't understand why our generation was spending so much money on an ephemeral good, something that was going to disappear. She began to research for her graduate school thesis, but what began as a few chapters evolved into a full-blown book. Four years later, Nestle called, asking her to pitch to their executive committee. As millennials come of age, large food companies are beginning to look for the best ways to appeal and market to them. That was when Eve realized there was a business purpose to her research—one that she hadn't been aware of initially—and her entire career trajectory changed.

I was in awe. How had she managed to turn a passion project into a full-blown, self-started business? Eve attributed her success to one main reason. "From what I can tell, I remain more of an encyclopedia for this topic than anyone else I've ever met." Her extensive knowledge of such a niche subject—millennial food culture—gave her credibility, and the rest came with time and experience.

While she was confident in her research and consulting skills, which had been honed through years of journalistic interviewing and academic analysis, it took practice to learn to speak with more authority and to become more confident in the business aspects of her job. Eve retained humility. I could hear it in the way she spoke, but I could also hear her passion, dedication, and ambition shine through her stories and the explanations of her research. For me, she will always remain an inspiration: someone who was able to channel her curiosity and passion for millennial food culture into a successful business model that simultaneously fulfilled a market opportunity and allowed her to pursue her passions.

PART III

TRENDS, FADS, AND THE BFLR METHOD

CHAPTER 8

FADS VERSUS TRENDS

———

I love listening to Blue Apron's recently launched Why We Eat What We Eat Podcast as I walk to and from work. Their story on the rise of kale helped explain the recent exponential growth of food fads and food trends.

Everything they were saying about kale seemed to make sense. It was versatile, easy to grow, easy to use, full of healthy nutrients. I was thinking, *Boom. A perfect example of a successful food fad.* Then I heard host Cathy Erway say, "We'll know kale has arrived when we stop talking about it."

I was confused, panicked even. Wasn't I writing a book about all these food fads because no one seemed to be able to stop talking about them? Had she managed to dismantle the entire theory of my book in one sentence?

I puzzled over this during the rest of my walk to the office and then again on the way back. The more I thought about what Cathy had said, the closer I came to realizing that she might have a point. When I hear the words "food fad," Instagram photos of sushi bagels, "yolk porn," stacks of decadent gourmet doughnuts, and ice cream sundaes piled with candy, cookies, and drizzled in caramel sauce flood my mind.

Kale certainly did not fit into that category. Kale was not something the Instagram community fawned over. Rather, it is an ingredient that had somehow managed to creep into the menus of restaurants, the produce drawers of our refrigerators, and the pages of our cookbooks. Eight years ago, no one knew what kale was. Today, kale is a kitchen staple. It's on one in five menus. It's even served at McDonald's.

How had this happened and what differentiated a food trend, like kale, from a short-lived food fad, like unicorn food? I set out to find the answers. (Side note: for those of you who might not be quite as well-versed in the most fleeting and frivolous of food fads, *The New York Times* has defined unicorn food as "any food item jazzed up with dye or cute accessories like fruit cut into little shapes or mountains of pastel marshmallows," best exemplified by the sparkly, pastel-colored frozen lattes that Starbucks sold for approximately one week.)

Why We Eat What We Eat's first episode, "The Search for Big

Kale," offered some great insight as to what distinguishes a food fad from a food trend and what led to kale's success. David Sax, the author of *The Tastemakers: Why We're Crazy for Cupcakes but Fed Up with Fondue*, explained that usually when food becomes a trend, it's because it has had a moment in which the food no longer represents just something you eat but becomes a symbol for something else.

He calls this the "cupcake moment" and recalls the example of Carrie and Miranda sharing a cupcake in front of Magnolia Bakery on the streets of downtown Manhattan in *Sex and the City*. That single scene represented a shift in our attitude toward cupcakes. They were no longer representative of the confetti cupcakes you made from a box for your six-year-old's birthday party, but rather a cultural symbol of luxury, social status, class, and identity.

The fact that kale did not have a cupcake moment may be indicative of its long-term staying power. Sax argues that the big food trends are not the ones that we Instagram, but the ones that fade into the background. Kale crept into the food scene at just the right time. As the farm-to-table movement took off, farmers' markets began to rise in popularity, and people started to care about what they were eating and where it came from, kale gained currency.

It became "the sophisticated version of lettuce," Sax said,

explaining kale's status as a symbol of class, identity and politics. That symbol gained so much traction because it became accessible, it was easy to grow, it quickly became available in grocery stores, and it was versatile. You could bake kale chips, throw it into a hearty winter soup, sauté it on the stovetop, or use it as the base for a salad.

Once I saw the way kale had worked, I noticed other foods that seemed to have a similar path to prominence. Just as kale had replaced iceberg lettuce, chickpea flour was beginning to replace white flour, cauliflower was beginning to replace potato, extra virgin olive oil had replaced vegetable and canola oils, pink Himalayan sea salt had trumped your average white table salt, and sriracha had become as much a condiment staple as ketchup and mustard. I had noticed each of these trends individually and was struggling to identify the common thread that linked them all together. I wasn't even sure if there was one.

In fact, when David Sax said, "Creating a food trend is kind of like creating a hit song. There's no formula to it. You can try and try, and it just doesn't work," in an article for *Culture Cheese Magazine*, I started to get discouraged. Were these food phenomena really just results of a combination of luck and timing? To some extent, yes, but in the same article, Molly McDonough also stated, "There's one thing that seems to unite all successful trends: they strike a chord at the right cultural moment." She was absolutely right.

Fads can be new, crazy, bizarre combinations of food, and they are exciting but ephemeral. They inevitably fade out once the initial buzz wears off. Food trends on the other hand, have to meet certain conditions in order for them to succeed on a large scale. By virtue of being labeled a trend, they have already reached a certain level of growth and ubiquity. While ramen burgers, edible cookie dough, and pork buns would inevitably lose their luster, kale, cauliflower, and avocado all fit into the health food movement, the rise of farm-to-table dining, and the newfound emphasis on sustainable agriculture.

A bit further into my research, I had the opportunity to ask Brett Schulman, the CEO of Cava, and Todd Klein, a partner at the Venture Capital firm Revolution LLC, to name the key factors behind sustainable food trends as opposed to ephemeral food fads. Brett's initial reaction was to ask, "Did you say poke bowl?" with a sheepish chuckle and a knowing grin. As the owner of forty successful fast-casual Cava restaurants, he was aware of all of the happenings within the fast-casual food scene, failures included.

"Not all fast-casuals are created equal," he said, emphasizing the need to stay true to your company's voice, the need for a menu that encourages frequency of visits, and the need for a dynamic array of ingredients that make your customers feel good. He recognized that fads come and go, and smart businesses help incorporate them but are not dependent on them. Todd Klein reinforced those ideas, highlighting the distinction between a trend that is attention-grabbing and a trend that can be offered on a large scale. A food trend isn't going to last unless a nationwide business can be built from it.

For Mike Kostyo, a major part of his job is to be able to distinguish between food fads and trends. Mike is a Senior Publications Manager at one of the three largest food market research companies in the US: Datassential, which has the study, prediction, and analysis of food trends down to a T.

Datassential has created its own framework for predicting food trends, which the company labels the Menu Adoption Cycle, or MAC. This method follows food trends throughout their entire lifespan—from inception, where they first appear in fine dining, all the way to the final stage, ubiquity, where they have reached mass markets and are being sold on supermarket shelves. In total, MAC includes four different stages: inception, adoption, proliferation, and ubiquity.

The first stage, inception, is where trends begin. There has to be something authentic and original about the food—whether it's the flavor, preparation or presentation—that puts it on the menus of fine dining or small, independent ethnic restaurants. From there, the trend moves into the adoption phase, where it begins to expand through lower prices, simpler preparations, and methods of use. In the adoption phase, trends begin to appear in fast-casual restaurants and gourmet or specialty grocery stores, like Whole Foods or Wegmans.

The next stage is proliferation, in which trends are modified in order to meet the needs of the mass market and mainstream customers. In some cases, they are combined with already-popular menu items such as burgers, pizza, or pasta to increase the chances of success. During the proliferation stage, foods are sold at casual chain and quick service restaurants as well as in traditional supermarkets and mass merchandisers on the retail side. The fourth and final stage is ubiquity, in which trends have reached their maturity and can be found across the entirety of the food industry, in family restaurants, convenience stores, and drug stores.

"It used to take ten to twelve years for foods to move through the Menu Adoption Cycle. Now it only takes six," Kostyo says, explaining the increasing speed and growth of food trends today.

One of the questions Datassential gets all the time is: What's the difference between a food fad and a food trend? The major make-it-or-break-it factor that Mike Kostyo cited was the democratize-ability of a food item. Can it be used in a variety of places and offered to a wide range of people?

As an example, he compared unicorn lattes to sriracha. There are only so many places in the industry where unicorn lattes could be successful. Sriracha, on the other hand, is appearing all over menus—from main courses to desserts and cocktails. You can put it in sauces, drizzle it on top of practically anything, or eat it on its own. Whereas the unicorn latte was a seemingly twenty-four-hour, social-media driven food fad, sriracha developed into a trend that managed to infiltrate the food industry nationwide.

Food fads are often recognizable by a few factors. If a food starts to appear prolifically throughout social media or its adoption on menus rapidly shoots up, as opposed to a steady rise, this typically means it's a food fad. There is no overarching need for fads.

Food trends, on the other hand, are democratize-able, as Mike mentioned. A huge part of that idea is the capability of being produced on a massive scale. There has to be enough of an ingredient or a trend to be able to reach a nationwide consumer-base. Wild animals, for example, will never be food trends because there simply will never be enough of them to satisfy mass markets. Trends are often indicated by organic, restaurant-driven growth that satisfies a greater, more profound need that exists throughout the larger society.

Mike helped particularly in connecting the dots between

the different health food phases that Americans have gone through over the years as well as explaining where we are now. Datassential has broken these trends down into what they call "Healthy 1.0, 2.0, and 3.0." Healthy 1.0 was the "low-fat, low-calorie" phase, where everyone was concerned with eliminating the bad, "unhealthy" ingredients from food. Healthy 2.0 encompassed the rise of farm-to-table dining and purchasing organic foods. People wanted to feel good about what they were eating, be able to trust their food sources, and feel confident that there were no pesticides or artificial additives in their food.

According to Mike, "We're still in Healthy 2.0 a little bit, but moving toward Healthy 3.0," which is the functional food phase that I will highlight in particular in the Nootropics chapter. Healthy 3.0 speaks to the idea that people want more from their food. They want their food to do something for them like increase energy levels or keep them satiated for longer. "Some things that aren't necessarily good for you can still give you energy and consumers will consider those things healthy," Mike adds. He cites mixtures and powders like moon dust as a couple of upcoming trends, particularly among young millennial women.

While luck and good timing may play small roles in sparking a food trend or getting people to talk about it, it's clear that a combination of factors must be in place for a food trend to reach market ubiquity—to truly be a trend and not a fad. If a food coincides with a broader cultural movement, its chances of success are even greater. However, among millennials and the foods they're going crazy for, four attributes stand out as necessary components to the success of a food as a trend. Is it healthy? Is it versatile? Is it easy to use? And is it mass marketable? A food that can combine all four traits is destined for greatness as a millennial food trend.

I have used these attributes to rank a number of rising and current food trends on a scale from 1 to 5. The higher a food scores, the more likely it will be to achieve success among the young foodies of Gen Y and millennials.

THE BLFR METHOD

Benson Food Longevity Rating

	A	B
1	Attribute	Description
2	**Healthy**	Combination of: - Functional benefits - Traditional nutritional perspective - Evidence of health benefits - What's a 5? Kale. Qualifies as all of the above. You could increase your consumption of this two-fold and it would be great for you! - What's a 1? McDonald's fries. Little to no health benefit. Increased consumption of item is not recommended. Does not provide health benefits or fit well into a balanced nutritional diet.
3	Versatile	Can you use/eat/cook it in a bunch of different ways? - Does it combine well with multiple ingredients? - What's a 5? Sriracha. Can put it on anything. It's been included on menus in desserts, cocktails, and as a condiment. Great thing to keep in your fridge to dress up a meal. - What's a 1? Truffle oil. Yes, it's often viewed as a delicacy and people tend to fawn over it. But it's a powerful taste, and not one you can just add it to any meal

	A	B
1	Attribute	Description
4	**Easy to use**	- Requires low effort, skill, and expertise - What's a 5? Pink Himalayan Sea salt. Available at all grocery stores now (wide accessibility) and is an easy replacement of a kitchen staple. Makes table salt a little more interesting but can use it on almost anything! - What's a 1? Harissa. A red chili paste that is certainly gaining attention with the rise of Middle Eastern foods. However, it's difficult to find in most grocery stores, is time-intensive to make yourself, and can be delicate to add to recipes because its spice is powerful
5	**Mass Marketable**	- A combination of cost, wide-ranging appeal, and accessibility - What's a 5? Extra virgin olive oil. Affordable, wide range of prices. Can be found everywhere. Used often in cooking, ends up in everyone's kitchen. - What's a 1? Bulletproof coffee. Cost and accessibility restrictions. Too expensive and too difficult to find to ever be sold to mass markets. As it's more ahead of the curve, it won't appeal to everyone.

CHAPTER 9

NOOTROPICS

———

Bulletproof Coffee, Spirulina, Fish Oil, & Collagen

"Trends and innovation . . . that sounds promising," said Chief
Marketing Officer of Ben & Jerry's, Dave Stever, over the phone
as he perused his computer files. The list of food trends he
had to offer sounded endless: food trucks, cultural collisions,
instantaneous delivery, meal kits, and gluten or dairy-free to
name a few. But of all of them, the one he advised to keep my
eyes on was nootropics.

"Noo-what?" I interrupted instinctively. This was something I
had never heard of before. Dave was kind enough to explain
that the term nootropics encompassed a new family of foods
that have the ability to elevate both the mind and body. "Certainly among Gen Z and millennials, it's all about eating on

the go. Snacking is now the meal. People are looking for foods that give them more than just calories; they want functional benefits," Dave explained.

He was right, from LA to New Jersey, techies, bio-hackers, and health food enthusiasts were going nuts for ingredients that claimed to provide heightened mental capacities in addition to beneficial health effects. I discovered four "superfoods" on the rise that fell nicely into this category. It only takes reading their names to realize that they must be on the cutting edge of the food industry. Bulletproof Coffee, collagen, fish oil, and spirulina are not ingredients you'll find in your traditional cookbook.

BULLETPROOF COFFEE

Dave Asprey is the founder of Bulletproof Executive and creator of Bulletproof Coffee, the latest fad that has been sweeping food-forward cities like San Francisco, New York, and Seattle. Inspired by tea mixed with yak butter that he discovered while hiking in Tibet, Dave created a mixture of coffee, grass-fed butter, and Brain Octane Oil that he claims suppresses hunger, offers steady lasting energy, and heightens mental clarity. While the evidence of long-term effects has yet to be confirmed, each of the three elements of the beverage is associated with certain health benefits.

The Bulletproof Coffee beans are said to be of higher quality than average coffee beans because they are sourced from Rainforest Alliance-certified coffee estates in Guatemala and Costa Rica and the standards for sourcing and processing are higher. This is said to eliminate mold and other toxins from the beans. The Brain Octane oil helps to balance your hunger hormones so that you feel full for longer and also converts to ketones, which are used more efficiently by your brain than carbs or sugar.

In addition to creating a creamy taste, the fat in the butter slows the absorption of caffeine, which gives you energy for several hours. The combination of the ketones and the slow release of caffeine creates a lasting alertness. But the perks don't end there. When made according to Asprey's particular recommendations, unsalted, grass-fed butter or ghee only, Bulletproof coffee beans and Brain Octane Oil combined in a blender will result in an ultra-creamy latte.

Rick Rubin, a music producer, who recommended the coffee to Ed Sheeran, claims that it tastes like "crisp toasted rye bread slathered with lots of butter blended in hot coffee." That's the idea behind Bulletproof. You're supposed to get all the warmth and flavor that you crave from a normal breakfast, but instead of filling up on sugary carbs, you're beginning your day with healthy fats that will sustain your energy, balance your hunger hormones, and elevate your cognitive function.

I'm going to be honest. I'm skeptical. In fact, the more I read about Dave, the more worried I became that this guy was a total wack job. He's a member of the "quantified-self movement" and a self-proclaimed bio hacker, meaning he obsessively collects data about his lifestyle and habits to understand and improve his behavior as well as modify his exercise routines and eating habits to improve his health.

Maybe a little neurotic, I thought. But then again, who doesn't want to improve their health? And isn't our whole society moving toward massive data collection? Then I kept reading, only to find out that before his interview with a *New York Times* reporter, he "dosed himself with a cocktail of substances to enhance his cognitive function." He wears specialty glasses that he believes protect his circadian rhythm from the glow emitted by his phone's screen, and he claims that through the "Bulletproof Diet," he boosted his IQ by over twelve points and lowered his biological age. This was beyond neurotic. His bold claims beg skepticism, and apparently, I'm not his only critic.

Joan Salge Blake, a clinical associate professor of nutrition at Boston University, states in a *New York Times* article that Bulletproof coffee is a far cry from a nutritious breakfast. Her primary concern is the lack of carbohydrates, which are known as brain foods. To her, Bulletproof coffee is just another fad that has gained marketing success because people enjoy the taste, but there is no confirmed evidence of the weight loss and other health benefits.

Dr. Frank Lipman, an integrative doctor, agrees. He occasionally recommends Bulletproof coffee for its temporary mental benefits, all the while warning that the drink is not nutritious because it lacks protein and other vitamins and minerals. Marion Nestle, an author and professor of nutrition and public health at NYU, says, "The success of the dietary-supplement industry is best explained by wish-fulfillment fantasies," dismissing Bulletproof coffee as nothing but a marketing tactic that has successfully exploited consumers' desires for a new weight loss strategy.

Additional criticisms include the so-called higher quality of Bulletproof coffee beans, as most coffee companies these days already partake in wet-processing, in which coffee beans are washed and their toxins eliminated. Others attribute some of Bulletproof's results to a placebo effect; if you believe this coffee is going to satiate your hunger cravings and make you feel more alert, chances are you will feel that way. There is also a lack of data on the long-term effects of nutrient deficiency.

Bulletproof Coffee

	A	B
1	Quality	Score
2	Healthy	4
3	Versatile	3

	A	B
4	Easy to use	2
5	Mass Marketable	1
6	Overall BFLR	2.5

My take: Not buying it

My recommendation: I recommend Bulletproof Coffee to only the most progressive and risk-taking of us foodies, those who are looking for the scientific foods of the future, and those who have the discretionary income to spend on something that could just as easily turn out to be a food myth.

SPIRULINA

Spirulina has been around since, quite literally, forever. It is blue-green algae that grows naturally in oceans and flourishes in warm climates and alkaline water. It is sold around the world as a health supplement. However, until recently, it was impossible to provide fresh spirulina to the general public because of outdated, unsafe, and unsustainable growth practices and a consumer market niche that was too small. While spirulina is now available in the form of pills, powder, or flakes, it's important to buy from a trusted brand. The algae can be easily contaminated with toxic substances or absorb some of the heavy metals from the water in which it was grown, so ensuring that it was sourced reliably and securely is a major component of purchasing the rising superfood.

This tiny aquatic microorganism is rich in protein, vitamins, minerals, and antioxidants, and, as with many new food trends, has been lauded for a myriad of health benefits, the majority of which have yet to be proven. These include its ability to boost the immune system, its makeup of 62 percent amino acids, which makes it a rich source of protein, its ability to protect against allergic reactions, and even an ability to combat viral or cancer symptoms.

Although spirulina has been touted as a superfood by scientists and nutritionists alike, most of the studies have taken place in animals or test tubes, so its effects on humans are yet to be confirmed. Others warn that although spirulina contains a high protein content, you would have to eat it in large quantities to ingest the same amount of protein you would get from meat or other protein-rich foods.

Nevertheless, the World Health Organization considers spirulina the world's best superfood and people love it for its high iron content, ease of digestion, and ample amounts of micronutrients and antioxidants. It's often sold as a health supplement or energy shot in smoothies, health food snacks and drinks, and recently has been introduced as an all-natural food dye.

The one aspect that might cause potential hesitation or resistance from customers is its taste. Spirulina is somewhat known for its particular flavor—a slightly salty, seaweed-like taste. "Taste is everything," said Shizu Okusa, emphasizing the high branding that would be necessary to debunk the myth of spirulina tasting like seaweed. Ultimately, spirulina will have to overcome the flavor obstacle and appeal to a broader range of customers in order to reach market ubiquity.

Spirulina

	A	B
1	Quality	Score
2	Healthy	4
3	Versatile	4
4	Easy to use	5
5	Mass Marketable	2
6	Overall BFLR	3.75

My take: Still skeptical

My recommendation: If you're a big smoothie maker, and you're looking for that extra protein-packed punch to elevate your smoothies to the next level, go for it. Otherwise, save your excess cash for something your diet may truly be lacking.

FISH OIL

One of the stories I found most fascinating in Michael Pollan's documentary, *In Defense of Food*, was the story of Wonder Bread. It all started in the late nineteenth century, when roller milling was introduced. Roller milling allowed food processors to shake off the bran and the germ of the grain during the harvesting process, which they then fed to the cattle. They used what was left to create the soft flour that makes white, fluffy bread that lasts almost eternally on grocery store shelves.

Unfortunately, that same process by nature also removes the majority of the nutrients from the bread sold to American consumers. "While you made the flour last, you basically ruined it as a food source," Pollan says. White flour was one of the best things that could have happened to the food industry because one mill could feed millions of people for extended periods of time; white bread doesn't turn rancid like wheat bread.

People did eventually realize, however, the negative health effects of nutrient deficiencies. Once again, the food industry found a solution to their benefit. Food companies quickly realized that if they had eliminated the natural nutrients in foods, they could just as easily add them in. That began the vitamin craze of the 1930s. Old Wonder Bread commercials boasted protein, calcium, and Vitamin B in their neatly sliced loaves of soft, white bread, even though they had already eliminated the naturally occurring bran and germ of the grain. "Why do you need to add all these special vitamins to bread? Well, because you've taken them out of the flour," Pollan explains.

Health-conscious consumers now scoff at the idea of Wonder Bread being nutritious—the idea is so antiquated. But I couldn't help but wonder if we are falling into the same patterns again today. Will Americans fifty years from now be laughing at all of the crazy dietary supplements we believed would make us live longer, decrease heart disease, and fight cancer?

Fish oils strike me as the modern-day version of the vitamin craze of the early twentieth century. According to *The New York Times*, fish oil was the third most widely used dietary supplement in the US after vitamins and minerals in 2015. At least 10 percent of Americans supplement their diet with fish oil. Fish oil, krill oil, cod liver oil, and algal oil all contain Omega 3s, which are essential fatty acids that your body can't produce. You must consume them through foods. Omega 3s are found naturally in fish, particularly cold-water fatty fish like salmon, mackerel, and tuna; nuts and seeds like flaxseed, chia seeds, and black walnuts; plant oils like soybean or canola oil; and fortified foods like eggs, yogurt, juices, milk, and soy beverages. Omega 3s are associated with numerous health benefits such as reducing the risk of heart attacks and strokes, fighting inflammation, and supporting brain health. One would assume that fish oils, being full of Omega 3s, would produce the same effect. So far, that doesn't prove to be the case for two major reasons.

First, because fish oil oxidizes easily, the fatty acids can be easily damaged from exposure to heat, light, air or from sitting too long on a grocery store shelf. Second, numerous fish oil brands have been accused of selling fraudulent or contaminated supplements. In 2015, four national retailers, Walmart, Walgreens, Target, and GNC were accused by the New York State attorney general's office of selling these deceitful diet supplements. It turned out that four out of the five products tested did not contain the herbs that were listed on their ingredients. Instead they were filled with cheap substances from rice and houseplants. To ensure that you are even consuming real Omega 3 fatty acids, Dave Asprey, founder of Bulletproof, recommends that you look closely at a brand's quality testing and processing methods, such as freshness and purity levels, the manufacturing process, the heavy metal content, and EPA/DHA content (which are eicosapentaenoic acid and docosahexaenoic acid, two of the fatty acids contained in Omega 3s). Because there is no US government standard for fish oil quality, he also recommends going by the European Pharmacopoeia Standard (EPS) to ensure the quality of fish oil supplements.

Also, there has been little to no proven evidence to support the beneficial effects of Omega 3 supplements. While many dieticians encourage the consumption of fatty fishes and consuming Omega 3s in their naturally occurring food sources, many remain skeptical about the effects of Omega 3 supplements such as fish oil. From 2005 to 2012, at least two dozen studies of fish oil were published in leading medical journals. Every study except two found that fish oil showed no advantages when compared with a placebo.

Andrew Grey, an associate professor of medicine at the University of Auckland in New Zealand, said to *The New York Times*, "There is a major disconnect. The sales [of fish oil] are going up despite the progressive accumulation of trials that show no effect." Elizabeth Johnson, who studies the role of antioxidants in brain and eye health at Tufts University, also voices her hesitation, claiming, "These nutrients don't work in isolation. They work together." This means you can't just expect to take fish oil supplements and have them function the same way they would as if you had eaten a piece of salmon. Elizabeth's claim is reminiscent of Pollan's argument in *In Defense of Food*. Just as we can't artificially add the natural vitamins that we have stripped from the bread during processing, we can't just replace our fish, nuts, and oil consumption with a couple of fish oil pills every day.

"The science of nutritionism gets hijacked by the ideology of nutrition," Pollan explains. Nutritionism is what the food industry uses to show us all the bad ingredients they have eliminated from their products and all the good things they have added. Pollan sees it as a critical flaw in our comprehension of healthy foods, because the ideology encourages the belief that the nutrient is the sole key to understanding food.

Americans used to fear protein; now they crave it. In the early days of Kellogg's Corn flakes, Americans viewed carbohydrates as the golden breakfast solution. Now, health-conscious consumers tend to avoid carbs like the plague. As quickly as our food opinions change, the food industry responds accordingly. When we began to fear fatty foods, labels like "fat-free" and "reduced fat" began to saturate the market. Now that there's a pervasive fear of gluten, grocery stores are offering entire aisles of gluten-free foods.

The problem is, Pollan explains, that none of these movements actually lead to a decrease in consumption of the "evil" foods. They simply lead to an increase in consumption of others. His overall advice is to avoid the noisy labels and shop around the outside of the grocery stores, where the fruits, vegetables, and other whole foods are often found. "The quieter the food, likely the healthier the food," he proclaims. I'm beginning to agree.

Fish Oil

	A	B
1	Quality	Score
2	Healthy	4
3	Versatile	4

	A	B
4	Easy to use	4
5	Mass Marketable	3
6	Overall BFLR	3.75

My take: I'll wait

My recommendation: In line with that of spirulina. So far, no negative health effects of fish oils have been observed, so if you've got a little extra cash on hand, and you're looking to up your Omega 3 levels—especially if it's been recommended by a doctor—I say go for it. As for me, I think I'll stick to eating fatty fish for as long as I can before someone tells me that my Omega 3 levels are low.

COLLAGEN

As with many of the food trends that seem to be sneakily infiltrating our lives, I started to notice the incorporation of a protein called "collagen" into everyday diets via Instagram. Suddenly, my favorite Instagram accounts were posting hot breakfast shakes, health-conscious coffee creamers and healthy pancakes that included collagen peptides. I had no idea what collagen was, but suddenly it was appearing everywhere.

It turns out, apparently, that I had been living under a rock. Collagen has quite literally always been everywhere. Collagen is the most abundant protein in our bodies, and it is vital to the maintenance of our body's structure of various tissues and organs. It is found in our muscles, bone, skin, blood vessels, digestive system and tendons. It keeps our skin resilient and flexible, our bones and teeth strong, and allows our joints to move without pain by strengthening our tendons and ligaments.

Collagen also creates natural creatine, an amino acid that increases new muscle growth after working out. Creatine can increase the gain of lean muscle, decrease recovery time, improve cardiovascular performance, and reconstruct damaged join structure. Collagen was starting to sound like a miracle drug . . . I mean, what exactly couldn't it do? I wanted to figure out just how beneficial to your health collagen actually was, who was using it, and how they were using it.

I started with Vital Proteins, the most common brand that seemed to be popping up on the Instagram accounts and blogs of all the health gurus I follow. It turns out that Kurt Seidensticker, the founder and vice president of the company, had been an avid runner until one day his legs were in so much pain that he couldn't finish. "I remember getting home from a run one day, and it being so painful that I actually broke down crying, not because of the pain, but at the thought of having to give up running," he says in Vital Proteins' brand video.

That thought sparked him to look at his diet and begin implementing collagen peptides into his everyday foods so that he could continue to run. With an array of lemons, avocados, and kale spread out in front of him, Kurt whipped up a green smoothie, blending in some of Vital Proteins' collagen peptides powder. "Bodies every year after the age of twenty-five are less efficient at producing collagen, so you combine this deficiency in our diet, along with our body's inability to produce collagen, and you have what contributes to health issues and aging," he explains. Finding a way to reincorporate collagens into his diet was his way of counteracting the aging process and allowing him to continue to do what he loves—run.

So who else uses it besides the man who created a company that sells collagen peptides? "Our customers are marathon runners and triathletes, but they are also weekend warriors, those who just want to run for the weekend. They're interested in eating healthy and digesting their food well," says Kurt.

He appears to be right. While collagen peptides are largely popular in the world of sports nutrition, they are leaking into the mainstream market as consumers become increasingly health-conscious. The global sports nutrition market achieved revenues of $20.7 billion in 2012 and is expected to increase to $37.7 billion in 2019. But the sports nutrition market no longer pertains solely to high-performance athletes. Now, "lifestyle and recreational users have recently emerged as lucrative user groups for the sports nutrition market," claims a 2014 report on the growth of the industry.

With the combination of a rise in health-conscious consumers as well as consumers who are eating on the go, sports nutrition food and beverage items are becoming more common as snacks or meal replacements for those who are on the move. Many people take collagen supplements in hopes of improving the strength of their hair, nails, and skin. Collagen can improve skin function by enhancing the skin's ability to absorb moisture. The more hydrated skin tissue is, the less likely you are to see wrinkles or cellulite. Collagen has also been suggested to help bone and joint diseases like rheumatoid arthritis or osteoarthritis.

As consumers have latched on to collagen for its numerous health benefits, companies have created collagen powders such as soy, cocoa, and cappuccino collagen that can be easily blended with beverages. These flavors tend to help dilute the distinctive taste of collagen, which isn't necessarily so great on its own. Others recommend blending it with sucralose or stevia extract to improve the taste.

While the collagen craze certainly had me intrigued, I still wasn't sure exactly how to use it. Fortunately, multiple nutritionists offer insight into the different forms of collagen as well as how to incorporate it into your diet. From what I've gleaned, collagen comes in two forms—protein and peptides.

The protein is also known as gelatin, which is created through the slow heating of collagen in water in a similar way one would create a bone broth. It can then be dried and ground into a powder. While collagen protein gels when it's mixed with a cold liquid, collagen peptides, on the other hand, are more easily digestible and tend not to gel. They can be mixed into both cold and hot foods and liquids.

Because of their similar makeup of amino acids, both types of collagen will provide health benefits, although nutritionists typically recommend collagen peptides for their variability of use and ease of digestion. Furthermore, collagen fits into the long-term food trends because of its versatility of use. A variety of recipes to cook, drink, and bake now litter the Internet. People recommend mixing it into both hot and cold beverages, adding it to gravy, soup, or bone broth, and even using it as an egg substitute in baking. In terms of a trending protein supplement, I thought collagen definitely had potential.

At this point, I was almost convinced. It didn't seem like there was anything bad about collagen . . . but just like with any other "superfoods" and dietary supplements that had recently begun to dominate the food scene, I couldn't ignore a lingering skepticism. For all the talk spouted by food bloggers, nutritionists, or performance athletes was there really any scientific proof behind the health benefits of collagens? As with spirulina, fish oil, and Bulletproof coffee, the jury is still out. Many scientists and nutritionists who study the effect of foods on our health still believe that the best way to consume these proteins and antioxidants is through eating whole foods like fruits, veggies, and sources of protein, like meat.

However, the studies that have been conducted on diets of added collagen have produced overwhelmingly positive results. The results of one twenty-four-week study of student athletes suggested that the consumption of collagen among athletes reduced the pain that would otherwise negatively impact their athletic performance. In a separate study, results showed that collagens taken during periods of resistance training effectively heightened the increase in muscle strength. Of the superfoods I had researched, collagen made me the least dubious.

Collagen

	A	B
1	Quality	Score
2	Healthy	5
3	Versatile	5
4	Easy to use	4
5	Mass Marketable	3
6	Overall BFLR	4.25

My take: Why not?

My recommendation: Of the four superfoods discussed, I would be most likely to propose collagen peptides for general use. With its high content of protein and amino acids combined with its ability to dissolve in both hot and cold liquid, it offers health benefits at a high ease of use. The next time you're making a soup, a smoothie, or your morning beverage of choice, why not throw in some collagen peptides?

CHAPTER 10

LIQUID NUTRITION

———

Matcha, Kombucha, & Fresh-pressed juice

In a book dedicated to the study of millennial attitudes toward food, it may seem odd to include a chapter on what appears to be the exact opposite—drink. But the thing is, some of the items that seem to be ahead of the food curve—highly functional, convenient, elevating of the body and mind—aren't foods you chew and swallow, but drinks that you can grab on the go. These beverages all offer a myriad of physical and mental benefits, such as higher and longer-lasting levels of concentration, improved gut and digestive health, and a simple way to incorporate more fruits and veggies into your diet, all in portable and highly versatile forms. Each one has its own unique history of origin, but all three are continuing to rise rapidly in popularity. To give you a glimpse into the world of liquid nutrition, I'd like to introduce you to matcha, kombucha, and fresh-pressed juice.

MATCHA

For the longest time, my roommate had been going on and on about matcha. Unlike most teas, in which components from the leaves seep out into the hot water, matcha is made from green tea leaves that are ground into a fine powder, so that when drinking, you're actually consuming the tea leaves themselves. As a dedicated coffee lover, I was skeptical, to say the least. But she wasn't the only one raving about matcha.

In 2017, food market research company Datassential, announced that matcha had increased on menus by 90 percent over the past four years. In 2015, *Bon Appétit* called it "the next big thing in tea" and claimed that food Instagram accounts are now "as likely to snap a picture of a matcha latte, as they are a cappuccino." This is in part due to the increasing presence of specialty matcha cafés sprouting up all over the country.

At the spring 2015 New York Fashion Week, models were sipping on matcha shots backstage, and Gwyneth Paltrow was featured on *Bon Appétit's* foodcast, praising matcha as her go-to method for satisfying 4 p.m. hunger pangs. Needless to say, this stoneground green powder has locked down quite the celebrity endorsement.

My curiosity got the best of me. Why matcha? Matcha, it turns out, fits nicely into the growing health trend among millennials. It's been lauded for its antioxidants, amino acids, and sustained energy boost. An amino acid called "L-Theanine" is responsible for the calm but alert effect that matcha creates. With less caffeine and a slower release than your average cup of coffee, matcha offers a sustained energy boost without the jitters or post-cup crash of coffee. It also speeds up metabolism because of its high level of catechins.

"In the modern world, people don't want to just be successful. They want to be healthy in a sustained way," says Graham Fortgang, cofounder of Matchabar, in an article for *Bon Appétit*. So far, matcha is doing exactly that.

What people seem to love about matcha just as much as its myriad of health benefits is the do-it-yourself factor. Shizu Okusa, CEO and founder of JRINK, swears by the bamboo whisk she uses for her daily matcha shot. Dietician and founder of Nutrition Stripped, Mckel Hill, says that making a matcha latte is a staple of her morning routine.

Many matcha lovers enjoy the ritual of whisking the powder into the water as a meditative part of the process. Matcha is also customizable according to the form the consumer prefers. While the traditional method involves only boiled water and the traditional green tea powder, people often add almond milk, soymilk, or dairy milk according to their taste. And if the traditional drink is not for you, matcha comes in both ceremonial and culinary grades. While the ceremonial grade is used as the base for matcha-flavored drinks, the culinary grade can be added for flavor to almost anything: baked items, smoothies, and desserts.

The versatility, personalization, and health benefits of matcha have cemented it as a food trend. "The better-for-you health trend is here to stay, with many manufacturers looking to remain ahead of the innovation curve with next-level products that capitalize on functional health benefits and convenience," Datassential claimed in its 2017 Foodbytes report.

So, I have to admit, I was intrigued. I found myself in Starbucks a day before an exam, and decided to give it a shot. I ordered a tall green tea latte with soymilk, per the recommendation of my roommate. I was slightly apprehensive as I waited. I had asked for the drink unsweetened and knew from the two years I spent in Japan that traditional matcha has a strong, bitter, almost chalky taste . . . which probably doesn't sound too enticing, but truly, it is delicious. It just takes slow sips and some getting used to.

I hadn't tasted matcha since then, so I had no idea how my taste buds were going to react. What I had neglected to remember was that Starbucks mass markets to American consumers, the majority of whom would most definitely not be ready for a straight shot of matcha. So when I took my first sip of the Starbucks latte, I was pleasantly surprised at its creamy sweetness. My next thought, though? If this was what "unsweetened" tasted like, what exactly does "sweetened" mean?

My curiosity piqued, I Googled the Starbucks beverage. The primary ingredient in their green tea latte was not the stoneground Japanese tea, but sugar. There are twenty-four grams of sugar in a tall latte, Starbucks' smallest size. To give you an idea of how much that is, the maximum advised daily sugar intake for an average female, according to the American Heart Association, is twenty grams, which is approximately 5 percent of a 2,000-calorie diet.

Although matcha has been rising in popularity largely due to its health benefits, those health benefits can be masked by an overload of added sugar. As with many of the trendy health foods that food companies often exploit, buying matcha powder requires a special attention to its method of production, its added ingredients, and the company that produced. But the benefits of the pure stoneground powder had convinced me. I went home and searched the highest quality matcha brands on the market, found a bamboo whisk to go with it, and ordered both items via Amazon prime so that I could make matcha my own way. Yes, I was skeptical of the companies that were attempting to mass market matcha to

American consumers by diluting its true taste and adding sugar. But I was also intrigued by this new alternative to my regular cup of joe. After just a few weeks of swapping out my morning coffee with a combination of matcha, boiling water, and warmed soymilk, I felt ready to proclaim myself a member of the "Matcha fam."

Matcha

	A	B
1	Quality	Score
2	Healthy	5
3	Versatile	4
4	Easy to use	4
5	Mass Marketable	3
6	Overall BFLR	4

My take: Already a matcha-lover

My recommendation: If you're looking for a caffeine alternative and are open to non-traditional flavors, I highly recommend giving matcha a shot.

KOMBUCHA

One of the biggest trends in liquid nutrition is kombucha. An air of mystery seems to surround this fizzy, fermented tea drink. Almost every Kombucha article you'll find on the

Internet mentions the lack of evidence behind its health benefits. Yet many people claim that kombucha is a "cure-all" and has countless benefits, including improved gut and immune health, healthier digestion, weight loss, and the control of liver cell toxicity. The American Cancer Society went so far as to promote kombucha as a cure for multiple sclerosis, arthritis, baldness, intestinal disorder, insomnia, cancer, and AIDS.

In fact, one of the top-ranked kombucha brewers in the country, Health-Ade Kombucha, first began brewing it as a preventative measure against hair-loss. Vanessa Dew, her best friend, Daina Trout, and her best friend's husband, Justin Trout, had created an entrepreneurship club together. They had no idea what their product was going to be. They just knew they were going to create something. But then, Justin came home one day and said, "I'm losing hair as a twenty-year-old male. This is bad news." The three decided to brew kombucha as an all-natural hair loss product. They used SCOBY, which stands for symbiotic colony of bacteria and yeast, as the hair mask and created all sorts of combinations of kombucha and SCOBY, but none worked. Eventually, they reached a point of defeat. With no training in clinical trials or hair loss monitoring, they felt deflated.

But they weren't going to let all of their high-quality, freshly brewed kombucha go to waste. Vanessa decided they should take all the kombucha they had created, bottle it, sell it, learn from the process, and use the experience to move on to their next venture. As they began to sell their first batch, they learned as much as possible from each consumer. They asked what moved each consumer to buy kombucha as well as what they wanted from it. Eventually, they decided to stick with kombucha instead on moving on to another venture, and they were able to take the information they had collected to effectively grow their company.

Five years later, Health-Ade is brewing 100,000 bottles daily, fermenting 50,000 jars weekly, and have raised 1,000,000 SCOBYs overall. The company prides itself on its brewing method, which they claim is "second to none." They utilize glass jars, 2.5-gallon small batches, and fresh-pressed juice. All of this allows them to create "real food" in the form of the best-tasting, highest-quality kombucha.

At a point when Vanessa, Daina, and Justin were still trying to make it in the kombucha industry, Vanessa happened to be in a Whole Foods in Los Angeles. As she grabbed a bottle of Health-Ade off the shelf, a young woman, unaware of who Vanessa was, gestured toward the Health-Ade bottle and said "Oh my god! This stuff has helped me so much. You don't even know. It's the best one out there! You're making the right choice!" That moment was priceless for Vanessa. Hearing a customer give such unprompted, positive feedback was the reassurance she needed to realize that Health-Ade was making an impact, and she had achieved success.

Kombucha's success is indisputable. The global kombucha market is expected to grow at a rate of 25 percent between 2017 and 2022, with its annual sales in the US already exceeding $500 million. Over half of the twenty-five to thirty-four age group are kombucha drinkers. When I spoke to Vanessa, I had my own thoughts on the reasons behind its success. As a beverage, it is certainly unique, in both its sweet and sour flavor and its fizziness.

It's versatile because the flavor possibilities are endless. It's easily portable, so that you can drink it wherever, whenever. Consumers have the ability to make their own. And perhaps most importantly, kombucha has achieved a perception of being healthy, regardless of the lack of scientific evidence to uphold these claims.

I wanted to hear Vanessa's take on the popularity of kombucha. According to someone who has dedicated her life to brewing top-of-the-line kombucha, what makes it special? Why is it going to last?

Her short answer was, "I think anything that makes people feel good is here to stay." Vanessa mentioned kombucha's status as the "better-for-you" product, the healthy probiotics in kombucha that align with the health craze, and the fact that it's ready to drink on the go. But more than anything, she feels that kombucha represents the obsession with real food.

Customers now want to know where their food is coming from and how it's made. They want to be able to trust the company they're purchasing from. Its unique brewing method and dedication to making customers feel good allows Health-Ade to become one of these companies.

Vanessa intends to meet customers where they are by upholding quality and sustainability over Health-Ade's bottom line. Given the trends toward healthier alternative beverages, eating on-the-go, higher expectations of company transparency, and shared values, I don't see Kombucha, or Health-Ade, disappearing anytime soon.

Kombucha

	A	B
1	Quality	Score
2	Healthy	4
3	Versatile	4
4	Easy to use	4
5	Mass Marketable	2
6	Overall BFLR	3.25

My take: It's my favorite "treat yo' self" drink.

My recommendation: If you're open to trying something a little on the funky side and enjoy bubbly drinks, go for it. It might not be an everyday thing, but it's the perfect weekly pick-me-up.

FRESH-PRESSED JUICE

While many may still roll their eyes at the notion of a "juice cleanse," it appears that the overall concept of fresh-pressed juices isn't going anywhere anytime soon. I remember when I told my mom that I was going to try a juice cleanse for the first time. It happened to be smack dab in the middle of midterm season, and her first response was, "I hope you don't pass out from hunger during your exams!"

Needless to say, she was not a fan of the idea. And she's not alone. I'd probably be worried about anyone who *wasn't* skeptical of the idea of eating no solid food for three to five days. To be honest, I wasn't even sure I could do it. I had to ask myself if I was crazy for giving it a shot.

Three days later, I had survived. Besides the annoyance of having to get up to go to the bathroom every forty-five minutes, I had actually kind of enjoyed it. It was liberating not to have to think about my next meal or put aside time to cook or do meal prep. I definitely felt like I had cleansed my system. I had even lost a few pounds although I'm pretty sure

I gained them right back as soon as I transferred to solid food again. But there was definitely something to be said for the detox component of the juice cleanse. It was like hitting a reset button on your diet, so that you could start clean again.

While not everyone is sold on the idea of a liquid-only diet, the level of juice consumption in our everyday diets has spiked. Fresh-pressed juices have boomed into a $3.4 billion industry, *Forbes* reported at the end of 2016. Juices have experienced 1.6 percent growth since 2005 and are now served in 61.2 percent of all restaurants, claimed Datassential. Not only has the juice industry been rapidly expanding, but within the market, more exotic juices are spiking in growth. While orange, apple, and carrot remain the most popular flavors, beet juice has grown 95.3 percent in the four years leading up to 2016.

What does this mean? Fresh-pressed juice has moved from a limited, elitist health specialty to a nutritious alternative that can be found on grocery store shelves, on restaurant menus, in cocktail mixtures, and as a make-your-own-at-home staple. When Eric Helms, founder and CEO of Juice Generation, first began his company, his reach was local. It wasn't until Salma Hayek began to request Juice Generation drinks at her filming locations around the world that they decided to collaborate and take the fresh-juice delivery idea global. Juice Generation now conducts annual sales of over $30 million. "I've been doing this for seventeen years. Juicing is not a fad," Helms said.

Why has fresh-pressed juice been able to sustain its rise in popularity and solidify itself as a food trend? Well, it aligns perfectly with the dominant food trends of our generation. As Helms said, "Juicing allows you to get lots and lots of nutrition in a very concentrated way, so I think that's where our society goes. People want it faster, quicker, better, more."

Juice is the convenient alternative to consuming fruits and vegetables in their whole form, it is perceived as healthier than other snacks or liquid options, it is portable, and it keeps your digestive system running smoothly. Catering even further to millennial expectations of personalized food items, juices can be customized by combining a variety of ingredients, such as whey powder, bee pollen, wheatgrass, ginger, and blue algae, all of which are known to add nutrients and are part of the trend toward functional foods that elevate both our minds and bodies.

Lastly, juices can serve as a way to eliminate waste in your own home. They offer a method for cross-utilizing ingredients and using up unwanted items like outer stalks of celery, bruised or overripe fruit, herb stems, and citrus peels. Although it remains the most time-sensitive alternative, consumers are no longer required to order fresh-pressed juices to be delivered daily. With the one-time purchase of a juicer, they can create juices at home themselves.

Fresh-pressed juice

	A	B
1	Quality	Score
2	Healthy	5
3	Versatile	5
4	Easy to use	5
5	Mass Marketable	3
6	Overall BFLR	4.5

My take: If I had an endless supply of grocery funds, my fridge would be chock-full of juice!

My Recommendation: If you struggle to fit an adequate amount of fruit and veggies in your diet and you also happen to be pressed for time (if this doesn't apply to you, congratulations, you must be super human), I would absolutely recommend considering juices.

CHAPTER 11

KITCHEN STAPLES

———

EVOO, Pink Sea Salt, Sriracha, Kale, & Chickpeas

Now that we've covered some of the crazy, futuristic food items that probably haven't made it into your home kitchen yet, I want to take a look at some of the foods that probably snuck into your fridges and pantries without you even noticing they had suddenly become one of your food staples. For me? It was sweet potatoes. Suddenly, I was picking them up every trip I made to the grocery store. For my French host mother? Pink Himalayan Sea Salt was her new favorite ingredient. For my parents and their parents? Extra-virgin olive oil had become the cooking oil of choice. And for millennials? It's a tough call. I'm torn between kale and avocados. We wear T-shirts that have "Eat more kale" or "Beets don't kale my vibe" written across the front, but we are also being accused of being incapable of paying our mortgage because we spend too much of our income on avocado toast. What were the stories behind these foods? Why were they so popular?

TRENDY NECESSITIES (EVOO, PINK HIMALAYAN SEA SALT, AND SRIRACHA)

As mentioned previously, David Sax was the first person who made me consider that the biggest food trends might not be the ones that blow up on Instagram or are recommended by Gwyneth Paltrow, but that, perhaps, they are the foods that slid into our diets without us making a big fuss about them. Extra-virgin olive oil, or more commonly known as EVOO, was one of his examples.

After some preliminary research, it appeared that olive oil started to gain popularity around the 1980s because of newly published medical reports on its health benefits and the introduction of Tuscan food into American diets. In the 1990s, olive oil began to expand from specialty stores like Dean and Deluca into regular supermarkets. It was still exotic, but it was beginning to reach mass markets. Between 1992 and 1997, the sales of extra-virgin olive oil in supermarkets increased by 73 percent and came to represent a third of all olive oil sales.

What was it that made "extra-virgin" olive oil so special? According to standards applied by the International Olive

Oil council, the term "extra virgin" applies to oils that have less than one percent acidity. Higher levels of acidity indicate oils that have been damaged or mishandled. The minimal level of processing of extra virgin olive oil also keeps acidity levels low. The olives are simply crushed. Beyond that, there is no additional processing. Extra virgin olive oil is also known for its greener color and stronger flavor.

Beyond its reputation for higher quality, extra virgin olive oil is also lauded for its myriad health benefits. In a study on olive oil intake and its relation to cardiovascular disease and mortality, the National Center for Biotechnology Information explained that, "The health benefits of the Mediterranean diet have been attributed to the high intake of monounsaturated fat, mostly represented by EVOO."

The Mediterranean diet has long stood as a type of gold standard for healthy nutrition and has been associated with reduced risk of cardiovascular disease, as well as longer life expectancies. The science behind the beneficial health effects of EVOO stem mostly from its high content of antioxidants, like vitamins E and K, as well as its fatty acids. Olive oil has been linked to anti-inflammatory and anti-bacterial effects, the prevention of heart disease and type 2 diabetes, reduced risk of stroke, maintaining a healthy weight, and the promotion of brain health (helping to ward off diseases like Alzheimer's). It is also associated with healthier diets. Studies have shown that a higher intake of olive oil is linked to an overall healthier diet.

Health benefits galore, it comes as no surprise that EVOO has become a kitchen staple. But as with other food items that have come to dominate large markets, purchasing EVOO requires special attention. Much of the olive oil labeled "Italian" doesn't actually come from Italy, but rather from Spain, Morocco and Tunisia. Often, after the olives are crushed and pressed, the oils are imported to Italy along with a variety of other oils like soybean, vegetable, and canola that are smuggled into the same ports. Once in Italy, all of these products are labeled "extra virgin" and branded "imported" or "packed in Italy." When tested, a whopping 69 percent of imported olive oil labeled "extra virgin" did not meet the standards of expert taste and smell. Purchasing olive oil involves another lesson in being skeptical of the food industry as well as doing research to ensure product quality. I would recommend finding a brand you like and trust, and sticking with it.

Extra Virgin Olive Oil

	A	B
1	Quality	Score
2	Healthy	5
3	Versatile	5
4	Easy to use	5
5	Mass Marketable	5
6	Overall BFLR	5

My take: Always in my pantry

My Recommendation: I'm betting you already keep at least one bottle of EVOO on hand at all times. If not, I'd say what are you waiting for?

As I mentioned earlier, olive oil wasn't the only ingredient that snuck into our everyday cooking routines. Pink sea salts are now all the rage. In a recent *TIME* article, Alexandra Sifferlin claims, "Pink salt is everywhere: in salt grinders, craggy-looking lamps, sunset-hued slabs designed for cooking steak and even in 'salt rooms' at spas."

Made from rock crystals from regions of the Himalayan mountains often in Pakistan, pink sea salt gets its combination of red and pink hues because it is minimally processed and therefore contains impurities, as well as certain minerals like magnesium, potassium, and calcium. Its popularity is due in large part to the health claims that surround it. Some argue that sea salt is healthier because it contains a higher concentration of trace elements. Others claim that because it releases negative ions into the air, it can help eliminate seasonal affective disorder, improve physical and emotional health, cleanse the air from pollutants, and ease respiratory conditions.

What does science say? Research has offered that while the salt's release of negative ions may improve people's mood, those effects are not definite. With regard to consumption of the sea salts, some people do report higher quality of taste than regular white, table salt, and while pink salt may contain more minerals, nutritionists agree that you probably won't get health perks just from eating it. The fact of the matter is that all salts are primarily made up of sodium chloride, and any differences in their mineral composition contribute more to color than to any change in nutritional value.

An author for the *Huffington Post* wrote, "Specialty salt purveyors, like so many other food companies, are playing into many consumers' belief that natural must mean better for you," and I have to agree on this one. While I consider myself an unabashed fan of the pink salt, it is more for taste and presentation than under any presumption of quality or health benefits. The reality is that salt doesn't really offer any nutrients to begin with. It's one of the ingredients in our diets that we need to regulate rather than increase. As an aesthetically pleasing garnish, I'm all about it, but as a functional food, I'm not convinced.

Pink Sea Salt

	A	B
1	Quality	Score
2	Healthy	3
3	Versatile	5
4	Easy to use	5

	A	B
5	**Mass Marketable**	4
6	Overall BFLR	4.25

My take: I like it for its looks.

My Recommendation: If you feel like changing it up from your regular old table salt the next time you're food shopping, pick up some pink sea salt to brighten up your dishes! The last condiment that I felt absolutely compelled to discuss is sriracha. This hot chili sauce was named *Bon Appétit's* Ingredient of the Year in 2009. It increased on menus by 80 percent from 2013 to 2014 alone and can now be found on the menus of national chains like Subway, Bruegger's and Panda Express. As of 2016, sriracha was still increasing on menus at a growth rate of 37 percent.

It has been combined with mayo and aioli to appeal to a broader audience and has even transcended its role as a condiment, expanding into the dessert menus of certain restaurants. Technomic, a large market research company based in Chicago, has even labeled the search for new international flavors and condiments by chefs and food developers the "sriracha" effect.

The famous sriracha sauce, a combination of chili peppers, distilled vinegar, garlic, sugar and salt, came from David Tran, a Vietnamese refugee who arrived in the US around forty years ago. After his arrival in the Chinatown of LA, Tran began selling his hot sauces to local Asian food spots and word spread rapidly. He came up with his business title, "Huy Fong Foods" after the boat that had brought him and 3,317 other Vietnamese refugees to the US after the Vietnam War. He now operates a 650,000-square-foot facility, and perhaps the craziest thing about his story is that he has never spent any money on marketing. His brand strategy focuses solely on working hard and doing things right. Clearly, it has paid off.

Sriracha

	A	B
1	Quality	Score
2	Healthy	3
3	Versatile	5
4	Easy to use	5
5	Mass Marketable	5
6	Overall BFLR	4.5

My take: Holds a place in my fridge

My Recommendation: If you're not a huge lover of condiments, you might be okay without it. But the sauce is so versatile that I'd recommend keeping a bottle in your kitchen. You'll be surprised by how much you use it!

KALE

The story of kale is a fun one to tell. What began as the adornment of iced seafood platters and was sold in the largest quantities to Pizza Hut for the décor underlying their salad bar. More simply said, what began as something no one had ever paid any attention to is now on one out of every five menus, is being eaten by Gwyneth Paltrow on the *Ellen Show*, and is written across Beyoncé's chest in her 2014 music video.

Kale is a superfood in more ways than one. Ten years ago, kale was on 0.7 percent of menus, and today, kale is on 25 percent of menus. It has even made it onto the menus of McDonald's, Starbucks, and the Cheesecake factory. In Datassential's terms, kale has reached market ubiquity. Six years ago, Eve Turow Paul didn't even know what kale was, and now it's a staple of her diet. In 2001, Robert Muller-Moore, better known as Bo, was screen-printing pro-veggie T-shirts with slogans like "Lettuce be" and "Feel the beet." When a farmer asked him to design a shirt specifically that said, "Eat more kale," Bo complied and assumed that would be the end of it.

But the next time he was selling at the farmers' market, all people were asking was, "Where's the greatest shirt of all time? The shirt that says 'Eat more kale!'" His business was so booming that he expanded to bumper stickers and is now credited, at least in part, with kale's rise to fame. Earthbound Farm, a company that sells salad greens in grocery stores, is now selling eight times the amount of kale they sold two years ago. So why, and how exactly, did kale explode within the food market?

Let's start with the facts. As Dr. Drew Ramsey states in his book, *Fifty Shades of Kale*, "Nothing is sexier than a sharp, happy mind atop a lean, healthy body. Few foods are able to deliver this promise like kale." He's not wrong. There are simply not many other whole foods that can top kale's list of pros. It's nutritious, containing more vitamins and minerals than almost any other single ingredient and certainly more than your average type of lettuce. It's cheap, it's versatile to cook with, it's easy to grow, its growing season is long, and it pretty much lasts forever. It will outlast any other leafy green you have stored in your refrigerator. Those aspects create a certain inevitability to kale's success as a food trend. But, the funny thing is, kale is lacking in one of the single most determining factors of a food's popularity—taste. It's bland, chalky, and not particularly flavorful. "It does taste like cowfeed."—*Eve Turow Paul, millennial food consultant* "No one takes a bite of kale and says, "Oh, wow! This is incredible. I want to eat this every day."—*David Sax, author of The Tastemakers* And yet, kale somehow managed to sneak into our refrigerators, onto menus nationwide, and into supermarkets as large as Walmart. What made it so special that people decided to forgive its bitter taste and make an effort to like it? In the first episode of Why We Eat What We Eat, host Cathy Erway attributes kale's success to one major factor. "Kale became a symbol of sophisticated eating at the same time that farm-to-table eating became trendy."

Her co-participants, who included Eve Turow Paul, David Sax, and Mike Kostyo, all came to the same general consensus. Kale had hit the market just as various food movements were taking off, like the trends toward locally sourced food, healthier ingredients, and farm-to-table eating.

Eve Turow Paul explained that its flavor profile, being chalky and bitter, led people to automatically associate kale with a more refined palate, which led to kale's being branded with a certain degree of food knowledge and sophistication. Eve describes it as "the more sophisticated version of iceberg lettuce," and David Sax likes to call it "the edible Prius or the edible Subaru," indicating how kale has surpassed its status as a type of lettuce to become a symbol of something much more politically or ideologically charged.

Both Eve and David agree that kale has come to represent far more than a vegetable; it is now a symbol of class, education, health, identity, and social status. "Eating kale is like a political statement saying that you care about food, nutrition, and farming," says Dan Bobkoff. For all its nutritional value, ease of use, and durability, the symbolism behind kale has played an equal role in its grand and continuously rising success.

If the story of kale and its evolution into a social currency wasn't fascinating on its own, there remains an element of mystery behind the marketing strategy that supposedly carried kale to ubiquity. While some attribute the explosion of kale to Bo Muller-Moore's famous "Eat more kale" T-shirts, others attributed its success to Oberon Sinclair, a young woman who runs a PR agency representing couture fashion lines. In her correspondence with Eve Turow Paul, she claimed to be the representative of the American Kale Association (AKA) and took credit for the marketing that led to kale's success.

But when Eve Turow Paul attempted to get in touch with the AKA, she found that there was no existing contact information listed. When she reached back out to Oberon Sinclair in confusion, all she got was radio silence. So Eve decided to contact the three largest kale farms in the US, none of which, it turns out had ever heard of the American Kale Association.

When she realized there was no American Kale Association, she reached out to Oberon one last time to warn her about going public with the story that would expose Sinclair's false claims. Oberon finally called Eve back, admitting that she made it up and had only done so because she wanted the world to know and love the vegetable. Eve wasn't so easily convinced. Only one winner seemed to be emerging from the saga, and that was Oberon Sinclair herself, who has declined to comment ever since.

Not so surprisingly, kale has managed to stir up quite a bit of drama—both good and bad. On the positive side, kale has become so well loved in Vermont that State Senator Anthony Pollina attempted to make kale the state vegetable, claiming that "It's very resilient, like Vermonters." And in addition to the Sinclair vs. Muller-Moore debate, Chick-fil-A decided to sue Bo because they claimed that his "Eat more kale" slogan sounded too much like their "Eat more chicken" slogan.

The rise of kale somehow managed to transcend the limits of the food industry and sneak its way into pop culture, celebrity gossip, and political debate. It might just be the defining food trend of our generation.

Kale

	A	B
1	Quality	Score
2	Healthy	5
3	Versatile	5
4	Easy to use	5
5	Mass Marketable	5
6	Overall BFLR	5

My take: I'm a proud owner and wearer of one of Bo's "Eat more kale" shirts

My recommendation: Go for it. Kale can be intimidating to

use and cook with at first, but you'll realize how convenient it is the more you experiment with it. Raw in a salad, roasted as a chip, or boiled in a soup, kale is an easy way to up your daily nutrients.

CHICKPEAS

I can't lie. I got pretty excited to write about chickpeas. As a lover of all things chickpea myself—hummus, chickpea cookie dough, chickpea pasta—I was pretty psyched to figure out what all the hype was about.

The chocolate chip cookie dough made from chickpeas by P.S. Snacks was probably the first thing that got me hooked on chickpeas. I was pretty stoked that I had finally found a guilt-free way to snack on raw cookie dough, and the fact that the founder of P.S. Snacks was a college girl not so different from me didn't hurt either.

In college, Nikki Azzara (Wake Forest University 2014) was a "gluten-free foodie, an avid runner, and a health enthusiast," which all led to the launch of her food blog, Slender Seven, on which she posted healthy recipes with only seven ingredients or less. She wanted to find a way to make her favorite desserts plant-based, nutrient dense, and healthy so that they could be eaten at any time of the day without guilt. Once her friends and family started demanding her recipes, she realized there just might be demand for her healthy treats. So she ditched the traditional career path to launch her chickpea and black bean-based cookie dough in stores. Today, her products can be bought online and are sold all over the Midwest and Eastern half of the United States. P.S. Snacks products are even available at Whole Foods.

You might be skeptical—healthy cookie dough? Impossible. Cookie dough made from chickpeas? Just plain wrong. "The cookie dough tastes just like the real thing (I swear I'm not biased), but is actually good for you," says Nikki in an interview with Birchbox, an online beauty retailer.

Having tried it myself, I'm not going to tell you that it tastes just like the real thing. That's simply impossible. If you go in expecting to taste the creamy, sweet cookie dough filled with the grains of sugar that you can feel between your teeth, you're going to be disappointed. You have to be ready for the slightly less sweet, slightly grainier taste that the chickpeas create. That being said, I have a huge sweet tooth, and the chickpea cookie dough satisfies it. It manages to be a healthy alternative to a dessert that actually tastes good.

When I say healthy, I mean it. P.S. Snacks lists ingredients online, and there are only eight of them: organic garbanzo beans, almonds, organic semi-sweet chocolate chips, organic cane sugar, organic virgin coconut oil, baking powder, pure vanilla extract, Himalayan pink sea salt. Yes, there's a hint of cane sugar and some chocolate involved, but the number one ingredient is chickpeas! And who doesn't love pink Himalayan sea salt?

Banza pasta is another health alternative that has taken the food market by storm, and another one of which, I may add, I am a huge fan. Banza boasts 25 grams of protein, 13 grams of fiber, and only 43 net carbs, compared with your average white pasta, which contains an average of 13 grams of protein, 3 grams of fiber, and 71 net carbs. Similar to P.S. Snacks, the number one ingredient (of only four total) is chickpeas. They make up 90 percent of the pasta's ingredients. The last 10 percent includes tapioca, pea protein, and xanthan gum. Did your eyes narrow when you read "xanthan gum"? Mine did too.

But Banza seems to be aware of its skeptical consumers and openly defines xanthan gum on its website. According to them, it is a non-GMO ingredient that is produced from the fermentation of a sugar to add volume. It's derived from corn and only makes up a very small percentage of the product. Upon further research, I learned that xanthan gum is a common FDA food additive that helps to thicken foods like dressings and sauces. While the FDA regulates quantity, xanthan gum in small doses is not considered harmful to our health.

I decided I'd risk it and the next time I decided to treat myself with a trip to Whole Foods, I picked up a box. I threw some Banza penne together with pesto, goat cheese, cherry tomatoes, and arugula, and barely noticed a difference. Just as P.S. Snacks seeks to provide a healthy alternative to a classic favorite, Banza claims, "We took a household favorite and made it even better, turning the pasta you love into the pasta that loves you back!" Both companies have been careful to retain flavor and taste even when swapping out traditional ingredients with healthier ones, and they seem to be doing all the better for it.

But even if I've managed to convince you to open your mind to chickpea cookie dough and chickpea pasta, there's still the lingering question: What exactly is so great about chickpeas? Well, according to Datassential, chickpeas fit perfectly into the latest health trend, or what they have deemed "Health 3.0." They are a functional food that is not only full of protein and amino acids, but also can be sustainably farmed so that they positively impact the environment. Banza also praises chickpeas for their lack of gluten and their low ranking on the glycemic index, and The United Nations even went so far as to name 2016 the year of the pulse, which refers to crops harvested for dry gain like chickpeas, lentils and beans.

Chickpeas have been around for a while, but their dominance in grocery stores and on restaurant menus is more recent. "Chickpeas used to be relegated to salad bars, often hidden in a pool of liquid, rescued by a slotted spoon and served as a nod toward healthful eating," says Katie Ayoub in her article "Chickpeas Go Chic." At one time, they could only be found on the menus of Middle Eastern, Mediterranean, and Indian restaurants. But recently, chefs, restaurants, and food companies have discovered creative ways to make chickpeas appealing to a broader market.

Ayoub touts hummus as the "bridge" to all other chickpea creations; its texture and versatility as a spread helped get more people on board. Now, chickpeas are found not only in hummus but falafel, salads, bowls and are beginning to be used as meat substitutes. Datassential claimed that chickpeas experienced menu growth of 290 percent in the decade leading up to 2015.

Ayoub attributes the exponential growth of these round legumes to three phenomena in particular. First, the affinity for vegetables that has been ever-increasing under the umbrella of the overarching trend toward healthier eating has led more people to search for plant-based options. Restaurants and food companies have responded accordingly. Second, she claims that an increasing demand for Mediterranean and Middle Eastern foods has caused people to rethink chickpeas, experimenting with new textures, forms, and flavor combinations, highlighting their versatility. And lastly, on a similar note, because of the rapid growth of food trends, menu development has increased drastically. Chefs are simply creating new ways to use chickpeas on their menu, whether it's in fries, falafel, salads, desserts, or on their own. Now, almost half of consumers are likely to order chickpeas in a restaurant, and this functional ingredient has extended beyond the walls of restaurants into the fridges and pantries of mass market consumers.

Chickpeas

	A	B
1	Quality	Score
2	Healthy	5
3	Versatile	4
4	Easy to use	3
5	Mass Marketable	4
6	Overall BFLR	4

My take: Couldn't live without my hummus.

My recommendation: Find a way to incorporate chickpeas into your diet—be it hummus or cookie dough! As a veggie that tastes good and is chock-full of protein, it's the perfect kitchen staple.

PARTING WORDS

———

This is where I leave you. I hope that having finished this book, you have gained a more holistic understanding of who millennials are, what led us to our current food habits, and how we are slowly but surely changing the food industry for the better. Maybe millennials don't have it all figured out. We are perhaps too fond of our phones and social media and some of our eating habits may verge on unhealthy; We haven't overcome the power of big business to undermine honorable efforts toward a healthier, more sustainable food system; And most importantly, we have yet to develop a system for nationwide access to healthy food.

Fortunately, I trust that you also tasted the healthy seasoning of hope and optimism that flavors this book and that these tastes lead you to believe, as I do, that the major millennial food trends of today—trends toward plant-based diets, locally sourced food, small food businesses, and transparent production processes—are genuine, powerful, and here to stay.

The faces and voices of the millennial food movement are both inspiring and fascinating. They've given us a better understanding of how to use certain tools, like technology, social media, and modern modes of communication, to improve our generation's food culture. And they've showed us past, current, and futuristic trendy food items, which you can decide to incorporate (or not) into your own life with help from the BFLR method.

Before I bring this book to a close, I'd like to leave you with some final advice—words to consider as you make future food choices.

MAKE FOOD A PRIORITY AND EMBRACE YOUR LOVE OF FOOD

Your body, your brain, and your mental health all rely heavily on the food you choose to provide to your body. Food choices are therefore important. Treat them as such. As there's little else in our lives over which we have unlimited, individual control, our diets beg patience and attention. Embrace your love of food. Try to block out all the other noise—the constantly dieting friend who stresses you out, your body-builder

Instagram accounts, or the Coca-Cola ads that tell you Olympic athletes thrive on their Coke consumption. Eat what you love. Eat for *you*. Don't let anyone get in the way of your love for food.

GROCERY SHOP SMART

Go back to the basics. Think "the fewer ingredients, the better." Seek out whole foods. Look for fruits, veggies, whole grains, and forms of protein before anything else. Buy from local farmers and brands. Buy organically, and avoid the middle of the grocery store.

EAT WHAT YOU ENJOY

Food should bring you joy, and I'm not talking about the way that sugars, salts, and fats set off pleasure centers in our brain. I believe that you can enjoy a healthy diet while still incorporating your likes and avoiding some of your dislikes. This goes hand in hand with moderation. I'm not asking you to convert to a paleo diet or to never eat another processed food in your life. I mean, who doesn't love a good, old-fashioned Oreo? So indulge every once in a while, but keep in mind that the more that your overall diet centers around foods like whole grains, vegetables, fruits, and proteins, the better shape you'll be in.

EAT AS MANY MEALS WITH FRIENDS AS YOU CAN.

Go out to restaurants with friends and family members. Host a weekly dinner or happy hour. Take a real lunch break to eat food with a colleague. No matter how you do it, share your food with others. Hospitality and social interaction are two of my favorite things about food. Nothing beats eating with family, friends, and the people you love. And sure, snap a picture of that oh-so-stunningly crafted plate in front of you, but then maybe leave your phone off the table for the rest of your night. Savor the meal. Linger in the accompanying conversation for as long as you can. Try not to worry so much about your next commitment. In a culture where everything is becoming virtual, online, and instantaneous, let's savor one of the few things we have left that's tactile, slow, and right under our noses: our food.

With that, I wish you the best of luck in all your future food endeavors. As for me, it's off to the kitchen. I suddenly have a craving for some avocado toast . . .

Eat well!

Sophie

ACKNOWLEDGEMENTS

—

First and foremost, I'd like to thank my professor, Eric Koester, for urging me to pursue my passion. It's not every day that a professor tells you to discover what makes you tick and then helps you publish a book on the subject. Thank you, Eric, for giving me the chance to discover my own stake in the food industry and for equipping me to be successful there.

Second, thank you to every one who participated in the creation of this book. Whether you took time to chat with me in person or over the phone, to read through my manuscript, to offer design ideas, or simply to tolerate my constant stream of food and book-based chatter over the past several months, I appreciated every single minute of it. This book couldn't have been published without you.

Lastly, thank you to the people in my life who inspired my love of food and encouraged me to step into the food industry. Joanne and Christopher, you have been both role models and sources of inspiration as I've watched Flour and Myers & Chang grow under your leadership. Mom and Dad, thank you for all of the delicious meals you have provided over the years, the recipes you've introduced me to, and the funding of my innumerable grocery store trips and restaurant visits. And Emma, Brittany, and Iz, thank you for all of the hospitality, friendship, new recipes, and yummy food you have shared with me this year—I will always look back fondly on our Thursday night dinners.

WORKS CITED

———

1. "Asian Honey, Banned in Europe, Is Flooding U.S. Grocery Shelves." *Food Safety News*, 29 Oct. 2012, www.foodsafetynews.com/2011/08/honey-laundering/#.WozwZFLMyt8.

2. Asprey, Dave. "Fish Oil Quality: How To Avoid Bad Fish Oils To Get The Best Omega-3s." *Bulletproof Exec*, blog.bulletproof.com/best-fish-oils-krill-omega-3-fats/.

3. Axe , Josh. "What is Collagen? 7 Ways to Boost Your Health." *Dr. Axe*, draxe.com/what-is-collagen/.

4. Ayoub, Katie. "Chickpeas Go Chic." *Get Flavor*, 5 Jan. 2017, www.getflavor.com/chickpeas-go-chic/.

5. Bilow , Rochelle. "Matcha Culture: Everything You Need to Know About the Next Big Thing in Tea." *Bon Appétit* , 14 Jan. 2015.

6. Blechman, Nicholas. "Extra Virgin Suicide: The Adulteration of Italian Olive Oil ." *The New York Times*, o https://www.nytimes.

com/interactive/2014/01/24/opinion/food-chains-extra-virgin-suicide.html.

7. Boyle, Brian. "Millennials Leading the Way in Emerging Food Trends." *Food Processing: The Information Source for Food and Beverage Manufacturers*, 11 May 2015, www.foodprocessing. com/articles/2015/millennials-emerging-food-trends/.

8. Bulletproof Staff. "How to Make Bulletproof Coffee and Make Your Morning Bulletproof." *Bulletproof Exec*, blog.bulletproof. com/how-to-make-your-coffee-bulletproof-and-your-morning-too/.

9. Calfas, Jennifer. "Millionaire to Millennials: Stop Buying Avocado Toast If You Want to Buy a Home." *Time Inc.*, 15 May 2017, time.com/money/4778942/avocados-millennials-home-buying/?xid=time_socialflow_twitter.

10. Cenicola, Tony. "Fish Oil Claims Not Supported by Research." *The New York Times*, 30 Mar. 2015, well.blogs.nytimes. com/2015/03/30/fish-oil-claims-not-supported-by-research/.

11. Charles, Dan. "Can You Trust That Organic Label On Imported Food?" *NPR.org*, 23 July 2014, www.npr.org/sections/ thesalt/2014/07/23/334073167/can-you-trust-that-organic-label-on-imported-food.

12. Cox, Lauren. "Spirulina: Nutrition Facts and Health Benefits." *LiveScience*, 6 Feb. 2018, www.livescience.com/48853-spirulina-supplement-facts.html.

13. Dewey, Caitlin. "A growing number of young Americans are leaving desk jobs to farm." *The Washington Post*, 23 Nov. 2017, www. washingtonpost.com/business/economy/a-growing-number-

of-young-americans-are-leaving-desk-jobs-to-farm/2017/11/23/
e3c018ae-c64e-11e7-afe9-4f60b5a6c4a0_story.html?utm_term=.
fc10d6087813.

14. Epstein, Chloe . ""Brain Freeze" Takes On a Whole New
    Meaning." *Chloe's Fruit* , 1 Nov. 2016, blog.chloesfruit.com/
    brain-freeze-takes-on-a-whole-new-meaning-d17ec1ac3f8.

15. Erway, Cathy . "The Search for Big Kale." Blue Apron / Gimlet
    Creative , 11 Oct. 2017, creative.gimletmedia.com/show/why-
    we-eat-what-we-eat/episodes/search-big-kale/.

16. Fabricant, Florence. "Pouring It On: Extra Virgin Oil as
    a Staple." *The New York Times*, 10 Sept. 1997, www.nytimes.
    com/1997/09/10/garden/pouring-it-on-extra-virgin-oil-as-a-
    staple.html.

17. "Fancy Food Show ." *Datassential Foodbytes*, 2017, datassential.
    com/Home/DownloadPdf?pdfFile=02-2017.

18. GAY, ROXANE. *HUNGER: a memoir of (My) body*. CORSAIR,
    2018.

19. "Global Market Study on Sports Nutrition: Revenues to Exceed
    US$ 37 Bn by 2019 End, Sports Drinks Continue to Fuel
    Market Growth." *Persistence Market Research* , July 2014, www.
    persistencemarketresearch.com/market-research/sports-nutri-
    tion-market.asp.

20. Greger, Michael. "HOW BIG FOOD COMPANIES AFFECT
    NUTRITION POLICY." *Forks over Knives*, 9 Feb. 2016, www.
    forksoverknives.com/how-food-industry-affects-nutrition-pol-
    icy/#gs.90KarrM.

21. Gunnars, Kriss. "Why Extra Virgin Olive Oil is the Healthiest

Fat on Earth ." *Healthline*, 4 June 2017, www.healthline.com/ nutrition/extra-virgin-olive-oil.

22. Guyenet, Stephen. TEDxHarvardLaw: The American Diet. Retrieved from: https://www.youtube.com/watch?v=HC20O0-IgG_Y

23. Hashim, P, et al. "Collagen in food and beverage industries." *International Food Research Journal* , vol. 22, no. 1, 8 July 2014, www.ifrj.upm.edu.my/22%20(01)%202015/(1).pdf.

24. "Home." *The Whole30 Program*, whole30.com/.

25. Hosie, Rachel. "How Instagram has transformed the restaurant industry for Millennials ." *The Independent* , 11 Apr. 2017, www. independent.co.uk/life-style/food-and-drink/millenials-restaurant-how-choose-instagram-social-media-where-eat-a7677786. html.

26. "How Much Is Too Much? The growing concern over too much added sugar in our diets." *Sugar Science: The Unsweetened Truth*, University of California San Francisco, sugarscience.ucsf.edu/ the-growing-concern-of-overconsumption/#.W07vB1LMyt9.

27. Hua, Karen. "Why Juice Generation and the Juice Cleanse Trend Have Survived So Long." *Forbes*, 30 Dec. 2016.

28. Hutkins, Bob, and Khem Shahani. "Kombucha: Trend or New Staple?" *International Scientific Association for Probiotics and Prebiotics*, 18 Sept. 2017, isappscience.org/kombucha-trend-new-staple/.

29. Iserloh, Jennifer, and Drew Ramsey. *Fifty shades of kale: fifty fresh and satisfying recipes that are bound to please.* HarperWave, 2013.

30. Kamp, David. *The United States of Arugula: how we became a gourmet nation*. Broadway Books, 2006.

31. Kasper, Lynne Rossetto. "Lentil Underground: An alternative to the industrial farming system in Montana." The Splendid Table. March 13, 2015. https://www.splendidtable.org/story/lentil-underground-an-alternative-to-the-industrial-farming-system-in-montana

32. "Kombucha Market Analysis By Flavor (Original, Flavored), By Distribution Channel (Supermarkets, Health Stores, Online Stores) And Segment Forecasts To 2024." *Grandview Research*, Sept. 2016, pp. 1–99., www.grandviewresearch.com/industry-analysis/kombucha-market.

33. "Kombucha Market Share & Trends Globally Will Reach $2457.0 Million by 2021: Zion Market Research." *Zion Market Research*, 28 June 2017.

34. Lappé, Anna. "Don't Sugar-Coat High-Fructose Corn Syrup." *The Atlantic*, 20 Sept. 2010, www.theatlantic.com/health/archive/2010/09/dont-sugar-coat-high-fructose-corn-syrup/63195/.

35. Leech, Joe. "10 Health Benefits of Spirulina." *Healthline*, 4 June 2017, www.healthline.com/nutrition/10-proven-benefits-of-spirulina.

36. Leite, David. "Dining Through the Decades: 100 Years of American Food." *The David Blahg* , 12 Feb. 2018, leitesculinaria.com/10348/writings-100-years-american-food.html.

37. Lucy Kennedy, Bill Kerr, Ted Gesing, and David Mettler. Netflix, 2018. Documentary

38. Martin, Simon. "Brand Cult: Huy Fong Sriracha Sauce. How a Hot Sauce Came to Rule the World. ." *Ceros*, 2018, www.ceros. com/blog/sriracha/.

39. Michael Shwarz. Netflix, 2015. Documentary

40. Mustain, Patrick. *Dear Consumers, Please Don't Eat Healthfully*. Patrick Mustain, 2018, patrickmustain.com/project/ dear-consumers-please-dont-start-eating-healthfully-sincerely-the-food-industry.

41. Nguyen, Andrea. "The Original Sriracha." *Bon Appétit* , 4 Mar. 2013.

42. Nordqvist, Christian. "Can Fish Oils and Omega-3s Benefit our Health?" *Medical News Today*, 20 Dec. 2017, www.medicalnewstoday.com/articles/40253.php.

43. "Olive Oil Health Benefits ." *Olive Oil Times* , Feb. 2018, www. oliveoiltimes.com/olive-oil-health-benefits.

44. Orlov, Alex. "People are mixing collagen into their coffee to prevent wrinkles — here's the verdict." *Business Insider*, 7 Mar. 2017.

45. Patel, Deep. "Food Leaders Take Notice: How Millennials Are Changing The Way We Eat." *Forbes* , 26 Aug. 2017, www.forbes. com/sites/deeppatel/2017/08/26/food-leaders-take-notice-how-millennials-are-changing-the-way-we-eat/#131d0faa7175.

46. Paul , Eve Turow. *A Taste of Generation Yum: How the Millennial Generation's Love for Organic Fare, Celebrity Chefs, and Microbrews will make or break the future of food.* Eve Turow Interior, 2015

47. Reece, Natalie. "How to Launch a Side Hustle: Nikki Azzara

of P.S. Snacks." *Birchbox*, www.birchbox.com/magazine/article/
launch-a-side-hustle-nikki-azzara-ps-snacks.

48. Rubin, Courtney. "The Cult of the Bulletproof Coffee Diet." *The New York Times*, 12 Dec. 2014, www.nytimes.com/2014/12/14/ style/the-cult-of-the-bulletproof-coffee-diet.html.

49. Ruiz, Michelle. "Instagram Feeding Frenzy: How 'Influencers' Are Changing the Food Scene." *Bon Appétit*, 11 Apr. 2016, www.bonappetit.com/entertaining-style/trends-news/article/ rise-of-influencers-ruining-everything.

50. Sakimura, Johannah. "Is Sea Salt Really Healthier or Just Overhyped?" *The Huffington Post*, 17 Nov. 2015, www.huffingtonpost. com/entry/is-sea-salt-really-healthier-or-just-overhyped_ us_563149efe4b00aa54a4ca8b4.

51. Sass, Cynthia. "7 Things You Should Know About Matcha." *Health.com*, 27 Mar. 2015, www.health.com/nutrition/what-is-matcha.

52. Sifferlin, Alexandra. "Does Pink Sea Salt Have Any Health Benefits?" *Time*, 28 June 2017.

53. Stack, Liam. "'Unicorn Food' Is Colorful, Sparkly and Everywhere." *The New York Times*, 19 Apr. 2017, www.nytimes. com/2017/04/19/style/unicorn-food-starbucks.html.

54. "Smoothies & Juices Drive Growth." *Nestle Professional*, Nestlé 2018, 1 Aug. 2017, www.nestleprofessional.us/trends/smoothies-juices-drive-growth.

55. "Spirulina." *University of Maryland Medical Center*, 2018, www. umm.edu/health/medical/altmed/supplement/spirulina.

56. "The Menu Adoption Cycle ." *Datassential* , 2018, datassential. com/Home/MoreResources.

57. Violi, F et al. "Extra Virgin Olive Oil Use Is Associated with Improved Post-Prandial Blood Glucose and LDL Cholesterol in Healthy Subjects." *Nutrition & Diabetes* 5.7 (2015): e172–. *PMC*. Web. 22 Feb. 2018.

58. Vital Proteins Staff. "What is Collagen? 7 Ways to Boost Your Health." *Vital Proteins*, 2018, www.vitalproteins.com/pages/ what-is-collagen.

59. Wachob , Jason. "Melissa Hartwig, Founder Of Whole30, On Addiction & How Hitting Rock Bottom Inspired An International Health Movement." *Mindbodygreen*, 15 June 2017, www. mindbodygreen.com/articles/melissa-hartwig-interview-on-whole30-drug-addiction-divorce-and-more.

60. Wells, Katie. "Spirulina Benefits: 7 Reasons to Try It (& 1 Major Caution)." *Wellness Mama*, 11 Feb. 2018, wellnessmama. com/4738/spirulina-benefits/.

61. "What is Kombucha." *Health-Ade Kombucha*, Health-Ade, 2018, health-ade.com/what-is-kombucha/?v=7516fd43adaa.

62. Whitler, Kimberly A. . "Why Word of Mouth Marketing is the Most Important Social Media." *Forbes*, 17 July 2014, www.forbes. com/sites/kimberlywhitler/2014/07/17/why-word-of-mouth-marketing-is-the-most-important-social-media/#7001c11554a8.

63. Wortham, Jenna. "You, Only Better ." *The New York Times*, 10 Nov. 2015, www.nytimes.com/2015/11/15/magazine/you-on-ly-better.html.

64. Zdzieblik, Denise et al. "Collagen Peptide Supplementation in

Combination with Resistance Training Improves Body Composition and Increases Muscle Strength in Elderly Sarcopenic Men: A Randomised Controlled Trial." *The British Journal of Nutrition* 114.8 (2015): 1237–1245. *PMC*. Web. 22 Feb. 2018.

65. "11 Revolting Things Government Lets in Your Food ." *CBS News* , CBS Interactive Inc. , www.cbsnews.com/pictures/11-revolting-things-government-lets-in-your-food/6/.

66. "5 Reasons the Kombucha Trend is Here to Stay." Auguste Escoffier School of Culinary Arts, 19 Apr. 2017, www.escoffier.edu/ blog/culinary-arts/5-reasons-the-kombucha-trend-is-here-to-stay/.

FEATURED FOODIES

———

The people I was fortunate enough to listen and speak to over the course of my research

- Eve Turow Paul, a Millennial food culture expert and consultant, author of [A Taste of Generation Yum: How the Millennial Generation's Love for Organic Fare, Celebrity Chefs, and Microbrews will make or break the future of food]{.underline}.
- Mike Kostyo, Publications Manager at Datassential, a leading food market research firm based in Chicago.
- Dave Stever, Chief Marketing Officer of Ben & Jerry's.
- Christopher Myers, the Boston-based restaurateur and co-owner of Myers & Chang and Flour Bakeries.
- Mike Brucklier, Director of Operations at Flour Bakery + Café
- Emily Luchetti, Award-winning pastry chef and cookbook

author; previous Chairperson of the James Beard Foundation Board of Trustees.

- Brett Schulman, CEO of Cava Group.
- Todd Klein, Partner at Revolution Growth.
- Vanessa Dew, Co-Founder of Health-Ade Kombucha.
- Chloe Epstein, Founder of Chloe's Fruit Pops.
- Anita Shepherd, Founder of Anita's Yogurt.
- Nekisia Davis, Founder of Early Bird Granola.
- Shizu Okusa, Co-Founder of JRINK Juicery.
- Andy Brown, Founder of Eat Pizza
- Samy Kobrosly, Co-Founder of Snacklins
- Justin Schuble, Instagram influencer @dcfoodporn
- Brittany Arnett, Co-Founder of Georgetown University Eating Society and Instagram influencer @toastedtable
- Emily Morse, Instagram influencer @new_fork_city
- Sarah Bellovin Goldman, PH.D. Clinical Psychologist at Georgetown University.
- Carol Day, RN, MSN, CNS. Direct of Health Education Services at Georgetown University

13720223R00115

Made in the USA
Middletown, DE
18 November 2018